BEHIND THE SMILE: MY STORY FOR HIS GLORY

BEHIND THE SMILE: MY STORY FOR HIS GLORY

My Story for His Glory

BETTY VIEHMANN RAYMOND

Acknowledgments

It is an overwhelming task to review an entire life and select the different events and scenarios that should be included. I prayed for Jesus to send in the help I needed. I knew this was His book and in His faithfulness, He sent in the "troops." I extend my greatest thanks to Him and to the following people.

My daughters, Carolyn and Maureen, my cheerleaders: They were the first "go-to people" for the initial input of this book. Thank you, Carolyn, my phone consultant, for my pictures, being my technology manager, and for your unwavering support and encouragement. Thank you, Maureen, for my inscribed pen, "I can do all things through Christ who strengthens me." Phil. 4:13. You supplied a Chromebook that enabled me to talk and print. Thank you for the encouraging symbols in my text as I progressed. You were awesome technical support, too!

My Thursday night church group: I appreciate your prayers and patience as you listened to my thoughts and questions throughout the progress of the book, and each of you always encouraged me with great expectation.

Sue: I appreciate your willingness and artistic contribution of your sketches. They were definitely inspired by the Holy Spirit.

Lisa, my book designer: This was a huge project that you accepted willingly when God tapped you on the shoulder. We have had a few glitches, but you have always been upbeat and encouraging. We learned together. This book would have been impossible without your expertise in publishing and formatting.

Kathy, Nancy and Vicki: Your final draft corrections and input were a great help and brought a level of excellence.

Lastly, I thank my husband, Howard, for living this life and loving me through my healing. You have been an anchor, a support, and the one who knows me best.

Dedication

To Aunt Ruth and Uncle Frank:

Much of the reflection of my life with you was seen through the eyes of a child and teenager. As an adult, I realize that without your generous hearts and sacrifices, I would not have grown into who I am. Even with the strict parameters, I see the Lord's hand in my life. You were humble, hardworking people that raised three sisters with very little material things. You gave us what we needed to the best of your ability to press forward in life.

With all my love and a grateful heart, I dedicate this story of my life to you, Aunt Ruth and Uncle Frank.

Until we meet again,
Betty

Preface

The only life one knows is the life you live. My life was one of dysfunction. But when you are young, you do not know that; it is normal for you. Through the years, many people had heard tidbits of my life and said, "You should write a book." Of course I didn't, but one day I heard the Lord say to me, "You are wasting your testimony." I knew then that He wanted it shared. My life is a regular life lived by many. The difference is that in the midst of all the dysfunction, Jesus knocked on my heart and I opened the door. Many deal with twisted emotions their whole life through no fault of their own. We are products of many things that form us. The purpose of this memoir is to declare that Jesus will come in and restore and untangle all the messed up emotions. He will lead and you will follow. It is that simple, but it often takes courage to face issues head on. His desire and plan for you is an abundant life and freedom to enjoy relationships. May our Lord show you through my life's journey how He leads, restores, and heals.

Contents

I

Early Childhood

Abandoned: having been deserted, cast off

"When your mother and father forsake you, the Lord will take you up" (Psalm 27:10).

"I will be a Father to you, and you will be my sons and daughters," says the Lord Almighty (2 Corinthians 6:18).

"Don't look at her, ignore her, she will be alright," Aunt Ruth said quietly, hoping it was true. There I sat, this cute three year-old in a mended and faded hand-me-down dress at a strange kitchen table. I did not really know everybody at this big eat-in kitchen. All eyes were on me and it was very threatening. I had blown out cheeks with tears welled up in my eyes, ready to break into a great outburst of crying. I tried to be quiet as I looked around this new, unfamiliar place. I was overwhelmed, scared, insecure, and seemingly all alone.

What could a three-year-old mind process? Absolutely nothing.

I was the youngest of five beautiful children, born in 1943 in Brooklyn, New York. My mother was a struggling young mom in her twenties, suffering from mental illness. My father abandoned us to be with a woman he later married.

I have no recollection of how, but we were brought to Glens Falls, New York. My grandmother's sister, Aunt Ruth and her husband, Uncle Frank, lived here in a very modest home. They had little financially, but took us in until someone could determine our fate. We were like pawns, moved from one place to another. As young as I was, I especially remember how we slept that first night. Uncle Frank used saw horses with boards across them; those were our beds. Heat was supplied by portable kerosene heaters upstairs and the coal furnace in the smelly, dirty, dark and scary cellar. We were together, but unbeknownst to us, this would be a very brief time.

Around two years old, before Aunt Ruth and Uncle Frank took me in, I was placed in a foster home. My sister, Madeline, would soon follow. She remembers the night when Social Services placed us. We were placed in a different home as our brothers, and as they drove away Madeline screamed, "Don't take my Freddy!" One memory Madeline had in the foster home was that if I did not eat the oatmeal she fed me, she was placed in a dark closet. That explains why, for years, I have never liked oatmeal. Some foster care homes only want an income from Social Services. This is one example of what conditions are like when that happens.

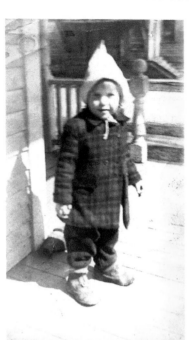

Betty, age 3, right before foster home
Haskell Avenue, Glens Falls, NY (1946)

My oldest sister, Barb, was passed from foster homes to relatives. She attended seventeen schools in her life. My two brothers, Fred and Ron, due to a lack of a foster home, were placed in a detention home for troubled boys. They were eventually placed on a farm in Washington County, New York. My oldest sister, Barb, arrived at Aunt Ruth's and joined Madeline and me at age 12. She was troubled, rebellious, moody and full of heart wrenching emotions.

When I was three years old, Social Services contacted my Aunt Ruth and asked if she'd be able to take care of me. I was suffering from malnutrition and emotional stress. She and Uncle Frank opened their home and their hearts to me. They had married late in life, were in their forties, did not have any children, and lived on a very low income. We lived three hundred feet within the border of West Glens Falls. For me, this was always a stigma for it was known as "Shantytown." It was a roof over my head and supplied the shelter and care I needed for now.

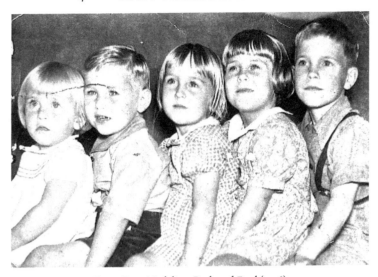

Betty, Ron, Madeline, Barb and Fred (1946)

There was a year gap in my early years that I don't really know who took care of me. My birthday was celebrated for a few years on September 27. I was shocked when Aunt Ruth told me we were celebrating on the wrong day. It was really September 21. I believe she discovered this from Social Service paperwork. Between having no baby pictures and an uncertain birthday, I felt completely insignificant. I felt unwanted and just simply *there*.

2

Life in the New Home

Insecurity: uncertainty or anxiety about one's self, lack of confidence

"I will never leave you nor forsake you" (Hebrews 13: 5b).

"My help comes from the Lord, which made heaven and earth. He will not suffer your foot to be moved. He that keeps you will not slumber" (Psalm 121:2-3).

That little girl sitting at the kitchen table was a bottle of pent-up emotions with no way to express them but cry. I lacked security, love, protection and was full of fear and anxiety. I was at the mercy of anyone that would take care of me.

Growing up in poverty is very difficult, especially the stigma associated with it. When school started, I realized other children had much more than I did. I don't necessarily mean material things, but they had an intact family. Other kids didn't seem to have the rollercoaster that comes with emotional dysfunction. In those days, family units were mom and dad. You didn't see many single parents, divorced families, or guardians - as my aunt and uncle were called. Mental illness was taboo, never spoken of aloud, and always discussed in a "hush, hush" way. It was scary and always brought shame on a family. It was often left untreated. I remember Aunt Ruth and my grandmother discussing my mom while talking quietly so I would not hear. *Shh, don't let anybody know!*

Second-hand clothes were our wardrobe. A neighbor ran a small shop of used clothing; it was the sole source of my clothing. It was a great incentive to work at an early age to actually buy something in style. I remember white bucks and a poodle skirt. I could be like everyone else. There were no extras like ice cream or gum as I was always concerned about finances. I worried at a young age; I never asked. That was life. One time I found a coin. I was probably five years old and walked by myself, a few blocks, to the corner store without permission. I bought gum and happily went home. My aunt saw me chewing my gum noisily. She said, "Betty, where did you get that gum?" I told her and that called for a big spanking with the back of a hairbrush. I had a strict upbringing. I learned. I obeyed.

My aunt had a dime bank. It was a little silver cylinder and you could slide one dime off at a time. As an adult, I began to realize how many times that little bank supplied our many needs. She was very frugal out of necessity. That supply was like the widow in the Biblical scripture 1 Kings 17:12 - 24. The widow was making a cake for Elijah, not thinking that she did not have enough for herself and her son. Elijah stated, "The

Lord said you will have enough." Like the widow, the dime bank was always replenished for needs due to our poverty.

Aunt Ruth sold greeting cards from house to house, often bringing me as I was just a little tyke. She sold Christmas trees in our front yard. She would make wreaths from running pine until her hands bled. She had a business mind and handled the meager finances well.

It was a challenge for them to take us in and bring us up, especially at their age. It was a lot of work, inconvenient, a huge responsibility and mostly thankless. They could have said no but by the goodness of their hearts, they kept my sisters and I together.

We had chickens and ducks, a garden, and would get our raw milk at a farm. The animals had names. One chicken, Junior, was pecked by all the others; he was our favorite. We tied a string on his leg so he could be identified and not chosen for our next meal.

It was not all fun and games. When Uncle Frank got angry with me, he would cuff me across my head. I often ducked. He'd say, "If it weren't for me, you would be in an orphan asylum." That just increased my insecurities which were already a big part of my young life. Or he would say, "You are going to be just like your mother." For me, that was one of the worst things he could say and had a tremendously negative impact on my life.

One Sunday after Sunday School, we arrived home to find Junior hanging on the line; he was the "chosen one." Shocked, I wondered, *Why would Uncle Frank choose that one?* We were careful to mark him with the tied string. I was angry, devastated and helpless. There was nothing I could do but accept this heartache. My wishes did not matter; it was heartless and cruel. Sometimes Uncle Frank would ask me to hold the flashlight while he was looking for the next chicken. Thankfully, Aunt Ruth would come to my rescue. Until this day, I still remember the distinct odor of plucking a chicken: the feathers sticking to my hands and the feel and smell of the warm skin. I thought, *Never again!* As an adult, I now realize Uncle Frank looked at our chickens as our meat, helping to feed all of us. However, as a child, my trust was broken again.

Aunt Ruth loved us, but with a controlling love. When she really got upset, usually easily, she would get "hysterical." That is what her doctor called it. One day Aunt Ruth, my two sisters and I were sitting at the kitchen table. She became very upset over something and slammed a glass milk bottle forcefully on the table. It broke and cut her hand badly, and she was bleeding profusely. The doctor arrived and tended to the injury. He also gave her medicine to calm her down. This had happened a number of times, these outbursts. We all became silent and watched. I nervously questioned to myself, *Did we cause this? Would they put us in the orphan asylum? Do we have to go to our mom?* Unanswered thoughts were floating through my mind. My life was different from my schoolmates. Most of them had a mom and dad and finances to make life easier. I certainly never shared anything about chickens or my mother or my aunt's emotional upsets. Deep inside I continually persisted, *No, hide behind that smile, all is well. Secrets, secrets!*

Aunt Ruth lived a fearful life. She would always anticipate something bad happening to us and held the reins tightly. We were not allowed to call her mom as she always said, "Your mother may come for you someday."

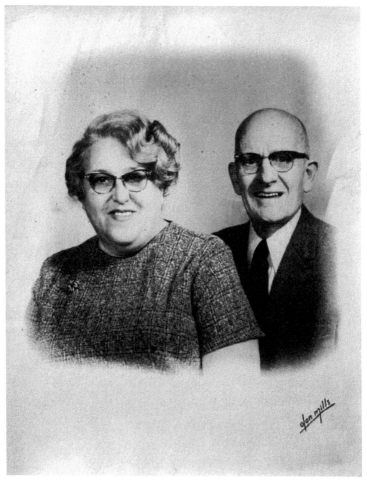

Aunt Ruth and Uncle Frank (1950)

That was not a comforting thought for me. I was afraid of my mother. We had no relationship. She always smelled like cigarettes because she smoked heavily. Her upper lip and fingers were nicotine-stained. She never tried to converse with me. No, I did not want to deal with her mental illness. My life was a roller coaster. Normal for me was always waiting for the "other shoe to drop."

Although we did not have much, we made our own fun. I "played store" with yard weeds. We had backyard picnics. I had a cat named Cubby, who was my favorite. I would dress him up and put him in my battered canvas carriage. It was quite a sight to see him jump out fully dressed and run away. I had an old bike and roller skates and would ride on the rough, cracked, bumpy sidewalks. These were good times in my world, almost carefree for a while or so it seemed. We joined 4-H and had fun at the meetings. We made different projects to be judged at the county fair, earning blue ribbons, which built my self-esteem. We made sewing projects, modeled at a dress review, and we did cooking demonstrations in front of a judge. All of these activities were a help in my development and were bright memories in my life. I could excel at something and be praised and acknowledged. I learned if I applied myself, I could do well.

3

My Brothers

Heartache: emotional anguish or grief, typically caused
by the loss or absence of someone loved

"He heals the brokenhearted and binds up their wounds"
(Psalm 147:3).

My two brothers lived about seven miles from Aunt Ruth
on a farm. They were well cared for and were used as farm
hands - plowing, milking cows, etc. We loved our brothers.
Aunt Ruth and Uncle Frank would bring my two sisters and
me to the farm for visits.

The adults would talk politics and we would go and play.
The barn was the most fun. Our brothers had very strong,
muscular hands from milking the cows every day. There were
plenty of barn cats who would line up at milking time so my
brothers could squirt milk right into their mouths. All the animals were named. Although I was the youngest, we did dangerous things. We rode bareback on Colonel, the horse, and

we rode in the hay wagon that almost disconnected as a horse ran away. We also played touch football in the thistles. One day we were laughing and giggling in the hayloft when a large beam fell on my sister Madeline's head! She was knocked unconscious. Perplexed, we thought, *What do we do? Do we jeopardize our visits? Do we tell someone?* We waited, and Madeline finally regained consciousness. We decided to never tell anyone, and we didn't. We treasured these carefree times away from the control at home. We could be kids, play, and actually feel that all was well in our world for a little while.

Periodically, our brothers would run away to our house and hide in our little woods. I don't know how they found their way throughout the seven miles. They would quietly call to us, and we would sneak out to play and have fun. It was unexpected and exciting! Each time they surprised us, my heart was full. *My brothers are here!* I would silently exclaim. It was wonderful being part of the secret that Aunt Ruth did not know. It was free time with our brothers, and they came all that distance to see us. It was a great adventure for them and an unplanned joy for us. In and out we went to see them all day long.

Barb eventually ran to the house and told Aunt Ruth. She called the police, for they were probably reported missing. The police arrived and we watched as they took them away. *Oh, why couldn't we be together?* I thought to myself. I am sure the police saw the sad situation, and they did not get in trouble. Eventually they were told if they ran away again, they would go to jail. It was dangerous and they obeyed. Again, I was helpless and torn seeing my brothers hauled away in a police car because they wanted to steal a few hours with their sisters. I was like a wave tossed in the ocean of life, good and bad emotions tossed up and down. I loved my brothers. They were older, but fun, and they included me. I missed them! *Put on that smile, all of us,* I thought. It did not matter.

My brothers' foster parents were Ma and Pa Brooks. We rarely had dinner or spent the night there. One day Ma and Pa asked my Aunt Ruth if we could go to the Schaghticoke Fair with our brothers. We were so excited! We would be going to a fair, riding in the back of a truck, but most of all, spending the entire day together having fun! The day arrived with a touch of a light sprinkle, but to us, it was full sun because we were so happy. All five of us piled into the back of Pa's old Ford truck with a tarp put on top of us to shield us from the rain. Ma Brooks had packed a picnic lunch for us in a very nice basket. We peeked inside. Much to my dismay, there were deviled eggs. My brothers led the way and started throwing the eggs at following cars. *Oh, so naughty of me to be part of this,* I thought. But, it was a memory I still remember fondly. The fair was awesome. We were tired children returning to the farm. I didn't want the day to end, and I especially did not want to say goodbye to my brothers. The time had come.

My brothers, Fred and Ron, stayed in touch as we grew up but never as an intact family. They had no interest in anything to do with our mother. Ma and Pa Brooks favored my father for some reason. Eventually, Ron moved to California to be near our dad, and my oldest brother, Fred, joined the army.

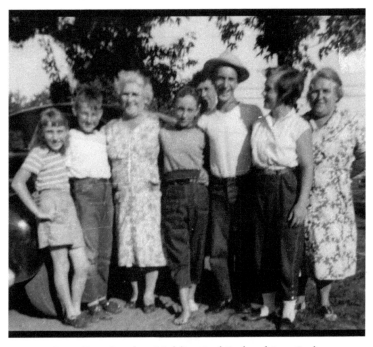

Betty, Ron, Grandma, Madeline, Fred, Barb and Aunt Ruth
West Glens Falls, NY (1951)

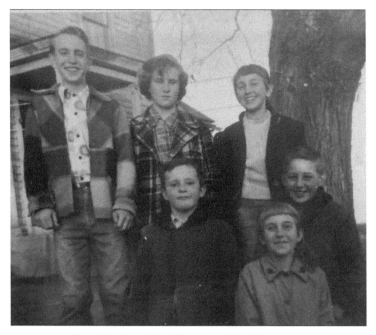

(Back) Fred, Barb and Madeline (Front) David, Betty and Ron
Ma and Pa Brooks Farm which is now Kelly's Feeds
County Line Road, Hudson Falls, NY (1953)

4

School Days

Respite: a short period of rest or relief from something difficult or unpleasant; hiatus, breather, letup

"The lowly he sets on high, and those who mourn are lifted to safety" (Job 5:11).

I attended Big Cross Elementary School, a small neighborhood school. It was five blocks from home, which was a long walk for me. My principal, Miss Riley, was a kind, caring, and wonderful lady. She would call me into her office and display a beautiful selection of clothes for me to pick out what I wanted; of course she helped. They were all the donations she had collected for her needy children. She never made me feel like I was needy, but I knew. She arranged violin lessons for me using a school violin. I found out in later years that my instructor was a famous violinist. A school violin stayed with me through high school. I enjoyed jacks tournaments, gym, music, hopscotch, and crafts. Elementary school was great!

I felt accepted and did well. No one ever knew the twisted emotions within me; inferiority, rejection, shame, and insecurity. I always had a smile. I never made waves for all seemed well to the outside world.

My Aunt Ruth was very supportive, but because of her constant worry and fear, she would never permit me to go to a friend's house to play. We three sisters had each other. That was enough she must have decided; we were safe at home.

5

Time for God

Confusion: lack of understanding; uncertainty, state of
being bewildered

*"Trust in the Lord with all your heart and lean not on your
own understanding; in all your ways submit to Him, and He will
make your paths straight"* (Proverbs 3:5-6).

A few blocks from my humble home was the West Glens
Falls Chapel. Aunt Ruth made sure we went every Sunday
to Sunday School and to church by ourselves. She never attended because she said she would cry every time. I think it
brought back her precious memories of Brooklyn with her
siblings and her childhood. She never stopped yearning for
Brooklyn. It was a small, little church body, one that loved
and totally accepted my sisters and me just as we were. I still
remember the hymns, "We've a Story to Tell to the Nations"
and "Standing on the Promises of God." Even then I knew
there was a God, but He was somewhere in the universe, very

removed from me. *Where was this wonderful God in my life?* I thought.

My pastor was a young man named Scotty Allen. He was married and had two children. We all loved him. He owned a plane and a motorcycle, was full of energy, and really related to the youth of the church. He loved to participate in our activities and spent much time with us. We would go midnight tobogganing at the Country Club. He arranged for an exchange trip to a wealthy church group in New Jersey. They had a gorgeous home and a maid, too. It exposed me to another way of life I had not seen before. This church body and youth group were an anchor for me, a safe haven of love, acceptance and growth.

I realize now that God had His hand on me. Yes, there was insecurity, abandonment, and my issues with my mom and dad. However, He gave me hope through my church family, my school principal, my siblings and my cat. *I will make it through*, I would frequently repeat to myself. I had a warm, humble home, food and love.

On Christmas Eve, my Aunt Ruth would go to the midnight candle service with us. It was a big deal to stay up past midnight. As she entered the sanctuary, she cried just like she said she would. It is a fond memory to this day and a precious time. We would get home late and very tired. We'd have a special treat and open our very few presents, an apron or something practical. Christmas was not about presents. We did not expect them. Santa Claus was not part of my life, nor was the Easter Bunny. I lived in the real world, not always full of everything a young girl wanted to be happy and secure. But maturity was reached at an earlier age than others. To this day

I love candlelight services and tear up just like my Aunt Ruth and for the same reason.

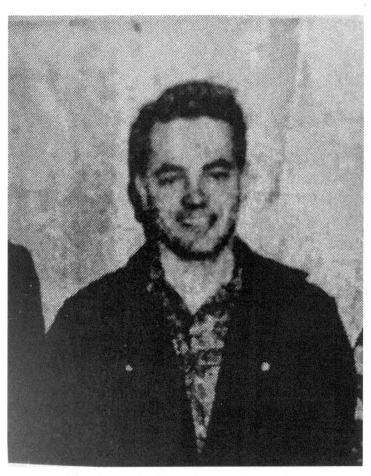

Pastor Scotty Allen He was the anchor for me and my sister and pastored at West Glens Falls Chapel on Main Street. (1959)

One Saturday, while at work, I received a message that my pastor, his wife, and children all died when his plane crashed.

I was devastated! My safe haven was pulled out from under me. I was on my own now, twisted emotions and all. I forged ahead in life with a smile. I stuffed my emotions and told myself, *I will do this. I can have a better life.* This was coming from a 16-year old girl dealing with a storm of emotions. I thought I wouldn't have to deal with anything while hiding behind the smile. Behind the smile I was terrified that what my uncle said was true; I was going to be like my mother. I resolved that never would be true!

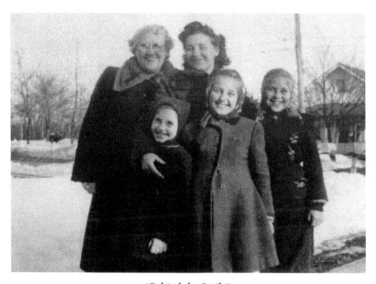

"Behind the Smile"
Grandma, Mom, Betty, Madeline and Barb
Aunt Ruth's house, West Glens Falls, NY (1949)

6

Enter Mom, Again

Shame: a painful feeling of humiliation or distress caused by the consciousness of wrong or foolish behavior

"Instead of your shame you will receive a double portion, and instead of disgrace you will rejoice in your inheritance. And so you will inherit a double portion in your land, and everlasting joy will be yours" (Isaiah 61:7).

Mom was always an emotional issue for me. Life would appear to be somewhat normal until my good intentioned grandmother would arrive with my mother from Brooklyn to visit us. I was seven or eight. The happiness of seeing my grandmother was totally dampened when I realized my mother was with her. It was stressful and confusing as a young girl. *Why was she not with us like a real mother?* I questioned. I was always told, "She is your mother. You must love her." I had no relationship with this medicated lady who spent much of her time puffing on a cigarette and staring. Mental illness had taken its toll.

One time mom and grandma came with two boys, one a baby. Their names were Jimmy and Paul, and they were born after me from a relationship with another man. Again, questions. My mind was overflowing with emotions, *Why does she have them and not us?*

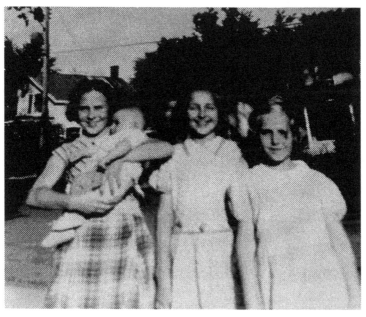

Barb (holding Paul), Madeline and Betty
West Glens Falls, NY (1950)

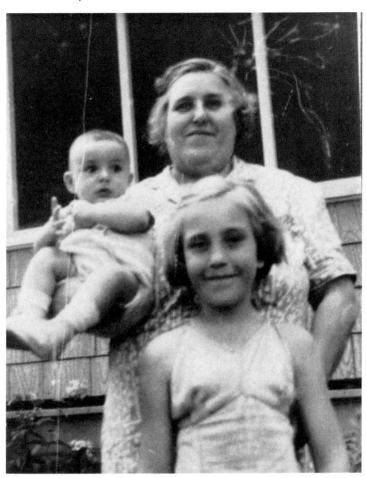

(Front) Betty (Back) Aunt Ruth holding Jimmy
Aunt Ruth's house, West Glens Falls, NY (1949)

Rejection hit hard, but of course I did not know. I was just there, not really participating, and mentally trying to separate from all of this. I was quiet and ignored her. I told myself I did not care and pushed feelings down. *My life will be better than this*, I thought. It had become my mantra. I never enjoyed those visits with mom. My classmates would ask me, "Where is your mother?" I would say she was dead. It was just easier. To me it was almost true. I had my smile; a great hiding place. I would not have to deal with anything while hiding behind the smile.

During one visit, my mother and grandmother's new husband had an altercation. My mom attacked him with a knife. I do not know what transpired to cause this. I remember hiding behind the sofa, scared and troubled. Bright police lights glared, attracting much attention from our neighbors. After much deliberation and many phone calls, they drove my mother away to a mental institution in Utica, New York. From there, she was transferred to Pilgrim State Hospital in Long Island.

At age 12, my faithful grandmother had arranged for my sisters and me to visit my mother. She was now at Pilgrim State Hospital in Long Island, a distance from Brooklyn. With her meager income, she still paid for a limousine to pick us up at her Brooklyn apartment and take us there. I dreaded this and did not want to see her. But I was told, "She is your mother, and you have to love her. Honor your father and mother." All of these thoughts were spinning in my mind.

A scene I have never forgotten was before me as we arrived. There was mom, thin, gaunt, and toothless, filing in a line behind bars on her way to see us. I anxiously wondered, *Was she going to be happy to see us?* Oh, the butterflies I had in my stomach and that awful feeling of dread. What does a 12-year-old do to relate to an expressionless woman? I did not understand at the time that the drugs caused much of this. What should have been a time of reunion, joy, and embracing was a time of fear, shame and dread. We went to a restaurant, embarrassed and self-conscious, putting on the "normal family look." People gazed; it was evident she was sick. I was very relieved to leave and escape from this painful encounter. This visit forever reinforced in my mind that I would not be like my mother. I would behave and adhere to the family motto: "Don't rock the boat."

After being released from the asylum, my mother lived as a caretaker for my grandmother. She should have been fully introduced to mainstream life but this was not the case. My grandmother was unable to be her advocate, and she became one of the many that fell between the cracks. The progress she made slowly diminished while she stayed in a Brooklyn apartment tending to the needs of my grandmother. After my grandmother's death, she was placed near her sister in a nursing home in Brooklyn, called Sheepshead Bay.

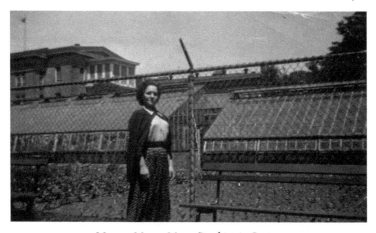

Mom at Mount Marcy Psychiatric Center
Utica, NY (1950)

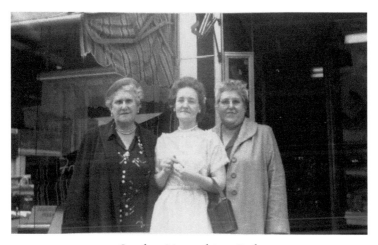

Grandma, Mom and Aunt Ruth
Pilgrim State Hospital, Long Island, NY (1955)

7

Teenage Years

Insecurities: deficient in assurance, beset by fear
and anxiety

*"But Zion said, the Lord has forsaken me and my Lord has for-
gotten me. Can a woman forget her nursing child, so she would not
have compassion on the son of her womb? Yes, they may forget, yet
I AM will not forget you. Behold I have engraved you on the palms
of my hands. Your walls are continually before me"*
(Isaiah 49:14 -16).

I was a "perfect" student. My smile covered all the "walls
of protection" I had erected through my life. This ensured
that no more hurts could come in. The real "me" wouldn't
come out. I was full of all the insecurities of life and its damage. I was quiet, well-behaved, and had a few friends who
never really knew anything about me. I did well academi-
cally. I played the violin in orchestra and sang in the choir.
Because we struggled financially, after school activities were

eliminated so I could go to work. My two sisters and I worked at the A&P grocery store on South Street in Glens Falls. We were very conscientious and dependable. Our boss loved us and gave us all the praise and acceptance we so craved. Due to our home financial situation, I had to pay board at sixteen. Surprisingly, I did not resent this. What I did resent was Aunt Ruth's strict rules. I was old enough to pay board and work but due to my aunt's controlling ways and fear, I was not allowed to date. My new pastor came to talk to Aunt Ruth and she lifted ALL restrictions; no more guidelines. While working at the A&P, there were many opportunities to flirt and date the packers. I loved this, but always put up those walls. Yes, let's have fun and go places, but I will not let you "in." Aunt Ruth had raised me with her fears so I still abided by most of the strict rules and expectations. Even though there was freedom, when I returned from a date, there was the clearing of Aunt Ruth's throat in disapproval.

While working at the A&P, I became very sick. I could not function like the hard worker I usually was in the past. I started to become nauseous and could not smell food. I was weak, tired, clammy and very thin. I laid in bed for two weeks, listening to everyone talk about food, either how delicious it was or what was going to be the next meal. The aroma of all cooking only made it worse. Aunt Ruth took me to a gynecologist. I am sure she thought I was pregnant (I was a virgin), but no diagnosis could be found. I returned to work, gaunt, still sick, but pressed through until I started to feel better. It took some weeks. Eventually after putting one foot in front of the other, I regained my strength. *What was that all about?* I questioned. My hidden emotions were trying to break forth, but I did not know this. *Smile, keep going*, I continually thought.

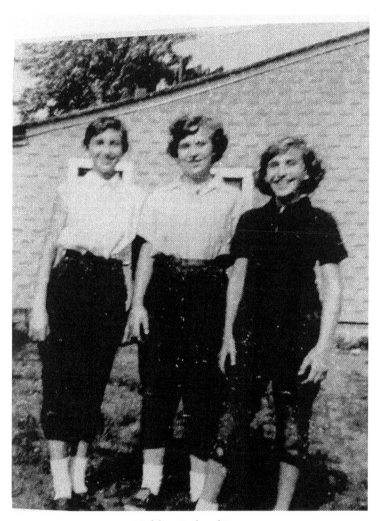

Madeline, Barb and Betty
Main Street, West Glens Falls, NY (1956)

In school I never felt I belonged, but felt on the outside looking in. It was not my classmates fault but my own troubled emotions; I felt inferior and never good enough. I did not realize I had troubled emotions as a teenager. I just lived life and did not try to figure anything out, just disappeared behind those protective walls. I needed freedom to be who I was. I did not realize I was trapped by these emotions.

I excelled in English, especially spelling. One time I was confused when I received a C grade. With all my courage, I asked my teacher why I received this lower grade. She looked at me and said, "As far as I can tell, you are not good at anything." I was shocked, hurt, and stood in disbelief. That comment fed into my unworthiness and shame. Words not only hurt, but are long-lasting and can cause much damage. I have never forgotten that moment.

8

Entering Adult Life

Failure: proving unsuccessful, stop trying

"For I know the plans I have for you, declares the Lord, plans to prosper you and not harm you, plans to give you hope and a future. Then you will call upon me and come and pray to me. I will listen to you" (Jeremiah 29:11 -12).

I was so proud of myself at my high school graduation. I chose the more difficult route and graduated with a Regents diploma. I even received a small scholarship. My next step was nursing school. I would be the first in my family to get a degree! I had to prove to myself that I could do it. Albany Medical Center School was the nursing school I chose. It was the most reasonable because nursing students were used as part of their labor force. It was known as a difficult school because work was a big part of it. Men's and women's surgical wards were my first assignment with less than five months of training. My dorm room was a single, with bars on the window, reminding me of my mother. My entire class was very downcast, discouraged, and many quit. I was to be capped in a month, and then it would be classes and working nights. Even though I carried a B average, I decided to quit. I could not handle it emotionally. I was overwhelmed and not prepared for life on my own. I had little finances, missed my boyfriend, and I was not a "party" girl so did not always join with other girls. Again, it was getting more difficult to hide behind the smile.

Quitting was foreign to me and truly a sign of weakness. But I did, and I now added failure to the list of looming emotions. Home, I went. *Now what?* I fearfully questioned.

Now at age 19, I returned to work at the A&P store. I was a skinny, stressed young lady, still presenting the image that I had it all together. But behind that confident smile was an unhappy girl who let herself down. I had great aspirations to obtain my nursing degree. After I quit, I became very discouraged. Entering nursing school, I thought *I'm worth something and I'll have a career.* Now all that was gone by my own doing. I was disappointed in myself, but was determined to push forward.

If I wanted anything extra, I had to save my own money. Working two jobs enabled me to buy my first car. It was a beauty, a 1956 Oldsmobile! It had lots of chrome, gray, with bright red upholstery. I loved to polish and clean it, take off, and drive. Freedom! I would drive to the countryside. I had a friend that lived in rural North Argyle. The idea that I was able to get behind the wheel with no agenda and just drive was exhilarating to me. I loved to drive!

My brother Ron came to live at Aunt Ruth's for a short time, even attending high school briefly. It was great having him there. One evening, I was on a date with a young man named Howard and I lent my car to Ron. While driving my car, he was involved in a severe accident. After dropping me off from our date, Howard heard the news on the radio and called me about the accident, leaving out many of the serious details. He took me to see my brother in the hospital. He had chest injuries and would be okay. I then found out that the other driver died and his son had a severe head injury. Howard proceeded to drive me to where my car was on display on a main street in Glens Falls. It was burned beyond recognition, tires and all. I was in shock, but displayed no emotion. Most everyone had heard about the accident on the news. When I went into my job to tell them I wouldn't be at work, I burst into uncontrollable crying. It was a release of all those powerful emotions. It all became real; the loss of life, my injured brother, and my beautiful car. Gone. The entire episode was very stressful. Standing by my car, I heard many negative opinions about the driver of my car. My brother was told by my lawyer to leave town. I was now an assigned risk according to the insurance company which increased my insurance payments. Because I still had to pay for my beautiful car, I was forced to drive a clunker that would literally lose its parts as I drove. I was embarrassed to drive that terrible looking, dilapidated car. All was settled by the insurance company and life went on as usual.

Howard was a mechanic, shy, and a very hard worker. We spent our date nights with three other couples square dancing. He loved country music, and this was so much fun. I loved being with him; I felt loved and secure. He often wanted to dine out, but for me, it was a trial because I had trouble swallowing and had no appetite. *Oh well, it is just nerves,* I told myself. While he was in reserve training, I would listen to "Soldier Boy" and the "Green Beret" on the radio. I'd think of him and wonder what he was doing. I would cry and enjoy my self-pity; not a sign of a well-adjusted woman.

During this time I worked as a teller in the local bank. It was a prestigious job, but not much pay. Being conscientious I did well, of course smiling, while I was waiting on customers.

9

Life Changes Quickly

Fear: distressing emotion aroused by impending danger,
evil, or panic whether real or imagined

*"For God has not given us a spirit of fear, but of power and of
love and of a sound mind"* (2 Timothy 1:7).

While sleeping one night, I woke up and I could not
breathe. My heart was racing, and I was cold and clammy. I
literally could not catch my breath. I was frightened and pan-
icked. I honestly thought I was dying. I frantically told Aunt
Ruth and she took me to the doctor. After some tests, he said
I was experiencing panic attacks. In the early 60's, this was
not common. There was no magical cure and no answer. That
night changed my life. For almost twenty years, I battled this
unknown enemy. Panic attacks consumed my life; either I was
experiencing one or anticipating one. It could happen any-
time and did. The only way to get through it was to escape.
My heart raced and I felt sometimes like I had a band around

my head. If in a store, I could leave, but driving a car or sitting in church, I was trapped. Even behind the teller window I was trapped. I dreaded all those situations but forced myself to endure them. It was exhausting. I was apprehensive being in a restaurant trapped at the table with all that food. I had difficulty swallowing. There was no freedom for my mind was always contemplating panic attacks. This was my secret, my torment, every single day. Attacks were ready to strike any moment like a rattlesnake. But I was a master by now at hiding behind my walls and smiling. No one knew. No one! I was NOT going to be mentally ill like my mother, as I was often told by my Uncle Frank. This battle was against an unknown adversary. It was a precursor to agoraphobia, but I did not give into it. *Push, push,* I'd tell myself. I did it to be a part of the mainstream of life.

Life goes on and I was still dating Howard. We became engaged and set the date in a few years. We were just like other couples dancing, drinking, quarreling, but really loving each other. I was convinced that marrying Howard would make me complete. That is an impossible assignment for anyone to fulfill. I had much to learn. We planned our wedding and due to limited funds, we had to pay all the expenses by ourselves, except for the wedding cake. Aunt Ruth was so proud to buy that for us. It was her contribution to my big day. I am sure that dime bank had a part in it, too. They really loved Howard and blessed our relationship. The wedding day arrived. It was a beautiful fall, sunny, crisp day on October 2, 1965. Of course, overshadowing everything for me was the anticipation of a panic attack during the ceremony. It was a large wedding party of thirteen with very beautiful fall colors. We were all set to become man and wife.

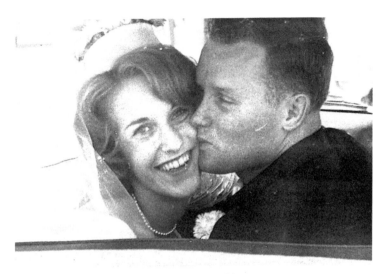

Betty and Howard's Wedding Day
St. Alphonsus Church on Broad St., Glens Falls, NY
(October 2, 1965)

My Aunt Ruth was assisting me; it was a very special time. All of a sudden I heard, "knock, knock" at the door. There stood my mother's sister, Aunt Grace, and with her was a surprise. There stood my mother ready to attend my wedding!!! *What???* Emotions swirled within my mind. This was not a surprise, but a disaster! This woman who I barely knew, who I was ashamed, and scared of, is here at my wedding on full display! There she stood in my pictures forever to be remembered. This was a true nightmare for me. I was shocked, ashamed, and trapped. With panic I thought, *What do I do?* The last thing I ever wanted was to have my mother here with all my friends. I ignored her. As an adult I know I was being selfish, but I just wanted to leave the situation. We stayed throughout the reception and then escaped on our honeymoon to live happily ever after. I left my mother, and I was so relieved to escape. Howard and I were together and happy, but not alone. "The Tormentor," as I came to call the panic attacks, was still with me. Our first year of marriage was turbulent. I thought all would magically be wonderful, but with so many unresolved issues, we had conflict. My security was always threatened by his buddies, for I saw this as a competition. We were headed down the same road as many young couples: partying, work, and living for ourselves. We lived across the street from a church and heard the bells toll every Sunday morning. I knew I should go but went back to sleep pushing the brief thought away. Jesus was knocking on my heart. I was raised to know God, but knew very little about Him. As a newlywed, I had many issues to deal with. I think He used those tolling bells to remind me there is more, like the fond memories of the West Glens Falls Chapel and all the fun and love there. He was seeking me.

The panic attacks came often. Adjusting to marriage, a new job, and a new town was difficult. My new home was in Herkimer, New York. It was a small, rural town that was much different than Glens Falls. I started immediately working at a bank as a teller again. I was on overload; getting to know a new job, new people, and not having a car. Howard used his company car. I was tending to meals and maintaining our small apartment, all while surviving the daily panic attacks. But no one would ever know it because I had my smile, my walls. No one ever knew *me*. The truth: I was scared, insecure, ashamed, fearful, and had a very low self-image. It looked like I had it all together. But, Jesus knew and so did I. *How long can you live hiding who you are?* I tried medication but that only complicated everything because now I was dependent on them. Life was closing in on me. Howard requested to be transferred back to Glens Falls as an insurance adjuster after one year. I was home again, settling in and working at the bank in a better position. The Tormentor followed me, always on my mind and in my life. It was agony and exhausting living a false life, fear of being discovered. *What am I to do?* I thought as I searched my heart. If I seek help, I admit I am mentally ill like my mother. I decided there was no way. I closed the door in my mind. Trapped!

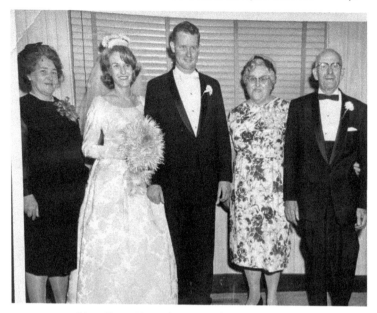

Mom, Betty, Howard, Aunt Ruth and Uncle Frank
Milfrank's, Route 9, Queensbury, NY
A sit down roast beef dinner was $5 per plate.

10

Honor Thy Mother

Responsibility: the state or fact of having a duty to deal with something

"Honor your father and mother, so that you may live long in the land the Lord God is giving you" (Exodus 20:12).

"You must continually honor your father and your mother which is the first commandment with promise so that it would be well with you and you would be long-lived on the Earth" (Ephesians 6:2).

During my adult life, I would see my mother in the nursing home once or twice a year. My husband's sister lived in Long Island. After visiting her, my husband would graciously take me to visit mom. These were "duty" visits for I was taught to honor my father and mother. It was always traumatic for me. I would go into this big room, filled with many smokers and find my mom sitting at a table playing cards. I would greet her and she would acknowledge me with no emotion and no joy in seeing me. She'd just continue playing cards. The visit was short for there was never much conversation. When I arrived, she often had her knee highs down to her ankles. Her clothes were too tight even though we sent clothes. I was ashamed to call her mom. It was so sad to see this woman's life.

The interactions we did have were awkward. I would leave and on the elevator burst out crying. Why? I didn't know. I was full of shame, rejection, and so many jumbled, negative emotions. *Jesus help me!* I would cry out. I have heard many wonderful things about this Jesus, especially in remembering my childhood hymns. *Was it true?* I continually questioned this in my mind.

There were many episodes with mom throughout the years. During this one particular trip, my sister Madeline and I, as well as her husband and three of our children, went to visit her. The children were young around 12, 14, and 16 years old. Madeline's daughters were the older two and my one daughter was the youngest. We greeted mom. We made her presentable and proceeded to a mall, a day to enjoy with her three grandchildren. That was *our* idea of a good day. After a few hours and quite a bit of walking, we were on our way back to the nursing home when she had shortness of breath. We dropped the girls off at the hotel telling them to not talk to anyone. It was scary for them, but we had no choice. By now mom had labored breathing and was not doing well. The weekend staff was sparse and I finally got someone to tend to her. "Oh," she said, "She just has a cold," and proceeded to put her to bed. I had that five months of nursing school and it was obvious she needed oxygen. The aide went 'very slowly' to locate some. I went to the desk and insisted they call an ambulance. We waited and then they told us they called the wrong hospital. By now mom had lost consciousness, which is called cyanotic. I said to the worker, "You are not canceling the ambulance!" The elevator doors thankfully opened and the paramedics had arrived. Lasix was administered, and by the time they transferred her to the ambulance, she was conscious. My sister and I rode in the ambulance. When we all arrived at the hospital, they did not want to admit her. I had to give my life story to the doctor so she could be admitted and placed on oxygen. That was a life threatening episode of congestive heart failure. The heavy smoking was not without consequences.

Meanwhile, our young teenage girls were alone in this hotel, which was recommended to us by a nursing home employee. We learned it was a hotel frequented by Playboy participants. It was a very stressful trip. Mom would have died had we not been there. I am sure our shopping trip contributed to it also. I returned home, emotionally spent, but thankful we were all safe. We left mom in the hospital, like a little child, but we had to return home. She was in God's care now; little did I know His plans.

11

Starting our Family

Grace: the free and unmerited favor of God, a divinely given talent or blessing

"But He said to me, "My grace is sufficient for you, for my power is made perfect in weakness. Therefore, I will boast all the more gladly about my weaknesses so that Christ's power may rest on me" (2 Corinthians 1:9).

In 1969, we were blessed with a beautiful baby girl, Carolyn. We were so happy! I worked at the bank part-time and had a born-again Christian babysitter. She was wonderful and so good for my baby. She lacked much in material things but was always so joyful, encouraging and content. With her sparse life I wondered, *Why does she have such joy and contentment?*

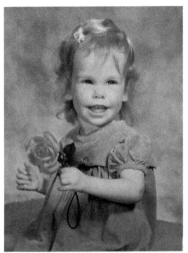

Little sweet Carolyn, age 3
Glens Falls, NY (1972)

When our daughter was two years old, she became ill with pneumonia. Just weeks after she came home from the hospital, her temperature climbed to 105 degrees and we rushed her back to the hospital. Our doctor could not find the cause and arranged for her to be transferred to Boston Children's Hospital immediately. The doctor gave us a choice: either go by ambulance or drive. Since we had little money, we started the 220 mile long trip. For four hours we traveled with our little girl in the front seat being sponged down constantly by me, hoping to bring down the temperature. When we arrived, she was admitted quickly as an emergency. Being a young mother, I did not realize how extremely serious this was. It could have been a multitude of diagnoses. My sister-in-law called and was so upset and said, "You just don't pray enough." These were hard words I did not want to hear, but it was true. I did not pray; God was nowhere in my life, so I thought. Those words stayed with me. The diagnosis was not serious and after three days, we returned home. I was in the middle of answered prayer and never acknowledged it. God was with us. I did not know it then but Jesus was knocking on my heart's door. He touched our little girl. This was just one of the ways He was caring for my family before I even knew Him.

Jesus never gives up; He continued knocking.

During this time, my Aunt Ruth became very sick. She had congestive heart failure and frequent hospital stays. My uncle worked until 10:30 p.m. so my sister shared caretaking duties. I would bring my baby and settle in. Aunt Ruth would lay on the sofa so sick and nauseous. We would watch television and the evangelist Billy Graham would come on. I would switch the channel to watch something that was not so boring. This routine went on for a long time until her final admittance into the hospital. One day I went to visit in the hospital and my sister-in-law was leaving carrying her Bible. Unbeknownst to me, she had presented the gospel message to her. Aunt Ruth asked forgiveness for her sins and asked Jesus Christ into her heart as her Lord and Savior. I was upset when I walked into the room and saw her crying. I now praise God that He led my sister-in-law to the hospital to see my aunt. I know I will see her again in Heaven. She soon went home to be with Jesus. Again, Jesus was knocking on my heart.

12

The "Key" at Last... I am desperate, Jesus

Desperate: feeling, showing or involving a sense of hopelessness that a situation is so bad as to be impossible to deal with

"I waited patiently for the Lord; He turned to me and heard my cry. He lifted me out of the slimy pit, out of the mud and mire; He set my feet on a rock and gave me a firm place to stand. He put a new song in my mouth, a hymn of praise to our God. Many will see and fear and put their trust in the Lord" (Psalm 40:1-3).

I returned to the Presbyterian Church after Carolyn was born. I was searching, looking for something, not sure what. I taught Sunday School. When a Billy Graham movie, "For Pete's Sake," came to our local theater, I asked my sister, Madeline, to go with me. Of course, the Tormentor, always uninvited, tagged along, too. I was desperate for anything.

Why not Jesus? It was an awesome and powerful movie! It spoke to my need for a savior and how much He loved me. This was a love that was absent in my childhood. I was still starved for love and acceptance. *Could this be true?* I thought with anticipation. The invitation was given to accept Jesus into my heart. We both walked to the front and talked to counselors who explained briefly about The Plan of Salvation. They explained that Jesus died for me to forgive me of my sins and give me eternal life. I opened my heart and said the prayer, not totally understanding all, but knowing I needed Jesus for sure. Little did I know this was the most important decision of my life!!!!

When some people accept Jesus, they are instantly on fire. Not me. Here I am, the same. I questioned, *Did anything really transpire when I invited Jesus into my heart?* I did not know much about the Bible and did not know that when you asked Jesus in your life, the Holy Spirit comes in. He makes you alive in Christ. Until then, spiritually, I was dead. Being a mom became most important, and my daughter, even more precious. Partying was much less appealing. I did start changing slowly from the inside out; attitudes changed, and I knew I needed to know more.

One day in my kitchen, I had a "light bulb" moment. It came suddenly for no reason; the thought that now that I have Jesus, I don't have to be like my mother. Hope at last! That was a comfort. At the same time I thought, *But how come I still have those panic attacks? Jesus, do you see me?* I rejoiced and wanted to learn more about this Jesus that knew everything about me. Jehovah Roi, one of His names, means "He sees me." Wow!!! I read in Psalms 27:10, "Though my father and my mother forsake me, the Lord will take me up." Here it was in black and white. The Lord was with me regardless of being abandoned by my mother and father.

In 1970 my husband built our little ranch home. We had our second daughter, Maureen, in 1973. She was a precious baby, and we enjoyed our family of four. Life was busy and stressful, and of course, I had wonderful times, too. It was fun enjoying my family and knowing the importance of a peaceful, happy, secure home. It's amazing how life went on, even in the midst of the battle with the Tormentor, who showed up daily.

I joined a Bible study with other young mothers. We met in a home, brought our playpens, and proceeded to study 1 Peter and 2 Peter. Interruptions were many. God blessed that sweet group of young moms who pressed on to learn more of Jesus, and we all grew spiritually. Now I was on the right path, but I had a long way to go. He was guiding me and holding me close, but still much had to be done, exposed, and healed. I knew the Bible says that God is the Healer. I wondered, *Why wasn't I being healed?*

One Easter there was a visiting minister at the Baptist Church where I now attended. I really liked his message; it was one of encouragement and enthusiasm. He was very charismatic. I started attending his church, an Assembly of God denomination. He soon built a new church and became legalistic leaving many of his beliefs and teachings behind. What did I know? It was a church family. It was safe and secure to have my pastor control everything. I was used to that. It was a non-denominational church where I met many great people, but really was not on the right path.

I learned some very good essential and foundational truths at that church, but always under the thumb of legalism. "Don't do this. Don't do that." The love of God was never emphasized. Control was emphasized. By now my youngest child was born, my precious baby boy, Daniel. God had placed in my heart to be faithful to church. I would load all three children every week and attend by myself while my husband attended Catholic mass. It was a great church body, but we followed the pastor more than God. I did not understand about a personal relationship with Jesus. There was more that I would soon learn. God did have plans for me, and I was in His hands. Praise the Lord that He was guiding me even though I was not aware of it.

13

Depression

Depression: persistent sadness, loss of interest, hopeless

"So do not fear, for I am with you; do not be dismayed, for I am your God. I will strengthen you and help you, I will uphold you with my right hand" (Isaiah 41:10).

Quite a while after Daniel was born, a slow and insidious cloud of depression crept over my life. These were not just sad days, but a deep, chronic depression. This time my smile and mask did not work. I wanted to cry. I couldn't drive, had no appetite, and was totally into myself and my depression. Of course with panic attacks, it is always about yourself. *What do I do? Jesus help!!* I cried out. I had three children and a husband to take care of, but I was in this black hole. I couldn't seem to muster any hope or energy. There was no pulling up the bootstraps. I was trapped, suffering greatly, but could not seek help. Stuffing emotions had taken its toll, and they were trying to get out. I felt trapped again. Even though God had previously spoken to my heart that I would not be like my mother, I found those thoughts rearing their ugly heads again.

Desperate, I went to my pastor for counseling. I presented my sad "woe is me" story. He listened and gave me a prescription: look up scripture for self-worth, read old hymns, and reach out to someone else in need. Also, there was one more thing, the big one!!! I had to forgive my father for abandoning me. I said, "What? Why would I forgive my father, a man I did not know and who left me?" I refused! I did not want to hear this, and it did not make sense to me. He quoted and wrote scripture for me to meditate on, specifically Matthew 6:14 and Mark 11:25.

Matthew 6:14 says, "For if you forgive men when they sin against you, your heavenly father will also forgive you. But if you do not forgive men their sins, your father will not forgive your sins."

Mark 11:25 says, "And when you stand praying, if you hold anything against anyone, forgive him, so that your father in Heaven May forgive you your sins."

I went home in my depressed state and read and reread the scriptures. It was very clear that I had no choice. I prayed and told God I was willing to forgive my father. I wrote my dad a letter and sent it to my sister who now lived in California, not far from him. I also found in Deuteronomy 32:10, "I was the apple of His eye." I was learning that a lot of what I felt about myself was not true! The truth was how my Lord sees me written in His word.

How did Jesus pull me out of this darkness? By reading His word and the message of the hymns, a small ray of hope arose within me. As I leaned on Him and followed the "prescription," I slowly climbed out. His word is light that shines in the darkness. This forgiveness was a very important part of my emotional recovery.

Do you need to forgive someone?

Dear God, Please give me the grace to unconditionally forgive (name), who has done me wrong. Give me strength to let go of all ill-will, the strength to forgive myself of my own failings and sins, knowing that you have already forgiven me. Free me of all anger, bitterness, hate and unforgiveness. Thank you Lord. Amen.

HALLELUJAH!!!!

14

Freedom from Panic Attacks

Trapped: a position or situation from which it is difficult
or impossible to escape

*"I will walk about in freedom, for I have sought
out your precepts"* (Psalm 119:45).

One of our church ladies had a life changing experience
with the Holy Spirit. She was a hairdresser. Many made appointments just to be near her and hear about all that had
transpired. She was glowing and changed. It was the beginning of a true Revival. The Holy Spirit started to reveal to a
core group of us that we had put our pastor on the throne.
This throne was the rightful place of Jesus. Many were healed
and saved, and many miracles took place. Church services
lasted until midnight; people were repenting and praying for
God's glory. We just wanted to stay in His presence.

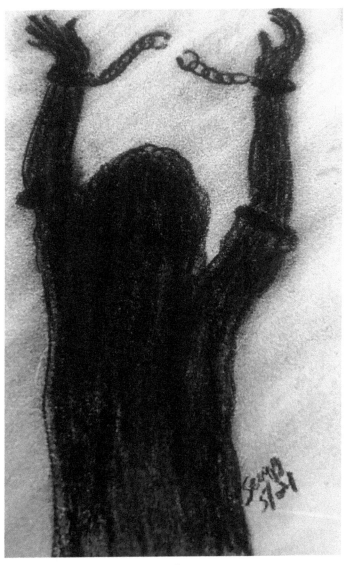

"Freedom"
Drawing by Sue Colucci

It was during the evening service that I went forward and asked for prayer for healing. No one knew why, but I knew. Jesus was the answer. It was between us, all His words I had repeated, all my prayers said, all my hope in Him. This was it; my only hope. The pastor prayed, and I sat down. There were no lights, no heat. I felt nothing different! The next day and FOREVER my panic attacks were Gone, Gone, Gone!!! Praise the Lord! He saw me and my desperate need. How faithful is my God!

Psalms 34:4 says "I sought the Lord, and He answered me; He delivered me from all my fears."

He said He was all I needed, and He proved it again!

15

Enter Dad

Forgiveness: the action of forgiving, pardon, absolution, formal release from guilt or punishment

"In Him we have redemption through His blood, the forgiveness of sins, in accordance with the riches of God's grace" (Ephesians 1:7).

"The Lord our God is merciful and forgiving, even though we have rebelled against him" (Daniel 9:9).

My Aunt Ruth hated my father with a passion. She had not one good thing to say about him and had no desire to see him, ever. One Easter, lo and behold, this big box arrived from my dad. We were so excited! *What could it be?* I imagined. We never heard from my father. As my Aunt Ruth opened it up, we gazed with big eyes at all the Easter candy. Wow, were we excited! We only got candy on Halloween, and now our father finally sent something to us. It was a brief moment of joy. We watched as Aunt Ruth slammed the lid shut and said, "This is poison!" *What? Our dad wants to poison us?* I sadly thought. Now we really knew he was horrible. Confusion, rejection and fear arose again. I questioned, *Why would he send poisoned candy?* He may have tried to contact us, but we never knew. The candy was thrown out. That is never the end of an emotional shock. Children do not know how to process these feelings. The emotions are often stuffed deep down, waiting to come out in other behaviors later. Even though the candy was not actually poisoned, as a child, I believed what I was told. This episode came to mind as I reached out to my dad.

After receiving my letter, my father contacted me by phone. He wanted to come to New York to see all of us. He must have been very nervous, too, with many questions spinning in his head: How would he be received? What did we know about everything? It was a short call, no frills, cautious, just setting a time for his arrival. I thought, *Did I really want to see this man who never contacted me and just left all of us?* The answer was, yes. I was now thirty years old and was meeting my dad for the first time that I could remember. A hope rose within me mixed with much apprehension. The time was set. It was 1974, and my middle child was a baby. I was extremely nervous when the day arrived! I was curious and anxious, anticipating meeting this man called "father." Again, I continued to question, *What do I call him? Where do I start? What is he like? Is he that no-good bum my aunt described?* I asked my oldest brother and sister to join me at my home because I did not know what to expect. Holding my baby daughter was a help and good distraction. He arrived. The awkwardness was heavy and filled the room. It lasted briefly. My first impression was that he seemed very nice. He was a big, gruff teddy bear. It went well, and my sister, brother, and I actually sat and visited with my dad, although we were all a little guarded. We purposely did not talk about the deep issues we all had; we did not want to rock the boat or hurt him. He related well to our children, and they responded to him. My dad had eight more children with his second wife. So now I had eight half brothers and sisters plus the two boys my mom had after I was born. I knew there were two sides to a story. The ice had been broken, and the visit went well. God was doing His work in my heart; the start of untangling my knotted emotions. I am glad God gave me courage to take the step to forgive my dad. It would take a while to find out who my dad really was, and God blessed him with 80 years of life. Another wall was falling down, a big one: abandonment. Thank you, Jesus.

Dad would call periodically. My sister and I eventually dared to schedule a trip to California to meet our eight half brothers and sisters. We had never flown before, so again, our anxiety was intense. We were so nervous that we took out life insurance for our trip at the airport. It's hilarious to think about that now!!

It was a stressful flight as I could not get past the psychological fear of flying. Both of us passed our food to a young man sitting in our row. He was ecstatic! During our layover, I requested non-smoking. We were kept off the plane until the end of boarding. We wondered, *Did we make a mistake?* When they called us, we were placed in first class! It was amazing! There was extra attention to every detail: pampering with a menu, real plates, warm hand towels, warm nuts and a hot fudge sundae cart. God, again, took care of my fear by blessing me with these extra comforts. This turned out to be a great memory. He let me know He was taking care of me. Just like He said in Psalm 27:10, "When your mother and father forsake you, the Lord will take you up." The hymn I sang in my childhood was true, "Standing, standing, standing on the promises of God my Savior; standing, standing, I'm standing on the promises of God." All of His promises are true.

We arrived and stayed with my oldest sister, Barb, who now lived in California. She had grown to love our dad. I am sure my new "siblings" were just as curious as I was. Dad had arranged for a fancy home cooked Asian meal. His second wife, Phyllis, was from the Philippines, and all my half-siblings resembled her. They were on their best behavior, not knowing much of our story at all. It went well. Again, we were a little cautious and distant, and we found out much about dad's life in California. Life there would have been very different from my life in New York. These children had also suffered poverty and hard times. My sister drove us to their homestead which was very run down, up a steep hill, and small for ten people. She relayed some of their stories. They had each other and had to make their own fun. They would slide on different things down the muddy hill. It was revealed that they thought we came from abundance. We were very different. We were always more quiet and subdued while they were always joking and very boisterous. Of course, we did not see that on this first visit. The stress ruled, and I am sure my dad put down the law. I now knew I wanted to pursue this relationship and start to know these new siblings.

There was a secret! My dad had a brother I didn't know existed. The fact came out when he accidentally mentioned his brother, Stanley. We let him know that we certainly wanted to meet him. Knock, knock! The door opened and a young lady named Sandra appeared, my cousin. She was gracious and friendly. Then, Uncle Stanley finally appeared. He was a big man, had a jovial face, and had a warm personality. After a short visit, we arranged a Mexico trip the next day with my dad and Uncle Stanley. We were so excited to drive into Mexico and spend the day with them! As we drove into Mexico we had so much fun enjoying all the unfamiliar surroundings. Dad gave each of us fifty one dollar bills to spend there. Dad and Uncle Stanley previously had a spat and had not seen each other in a while. This was a day of reconciliation and togetherness. Mexico was so different, and bartering was what we did. The car was full of mementos to bring home to New York, even a real Mexican piñata. That was something transporting it on the plane.

My dad had much regret in his life. He did try to reach out to us, but I am sure my aunt intercepted any correspondence. I remember a graduation card from my grandmother who I had never met. Dad did say, "Girls, I am sorry and I guess you want to talk about things. I did try to contact you, but your aunt prevented this." We did not want to ruin what had just started, a relationship with this man who was called dad by thirteen children.

Again, my faithful God, "Jehovah-Jireh," (God provides) took care of me. I was known as the "bump queen" because almost every trip I would get bumped and get a free round-trip ticket for my next trip. I would get to California at least two times a year and dad would come visit two times or more a year. The phone would ring and dad would say, "I will be at the airport at such a time." With no warning, we would just drop everything and pick him up. That was Dad. When he called from California, I would end the call and say, "I love you." His reply was a muffled, "Me, too and all that stuff." It was difficult for him, but eventually he easily said he loved me, loud and clear. He would be sitting in the recliner in my living room and I would crawl on his lap. There was no more awkwardness, but total forgiveness and love. We all looked forward to his visits for he was fun and all the grandkids loved him. He assigned nicknames as he studied each one. "Toe jam" for my daughter as he watched her clean out the sand from her toes after a day at the beach. "Booger roller," self-explanatory. "Moose," my tall daughter. "The gut," for me when I could eat anything and didn't gain weight. Finally, "the mayor" for my husband, for he kept it all together. These names only made him more endearing. My husband and he were sidekicks, working on our apartment houses or the project for the day. There was never a dull moment and we were making precious memories.

Dad often was with me for important happenings. He came to my daughter, Carolyn's, wedding and he came to be with my daughter, Maureen, before her scoliosis surgery. He was here when I was diagnosed with breast cancer, and he came to my son's most important football game. He also arrived for Carolyn's driving test. He was really very involved and interested in our lives and kept tabs on all of us. I always looked forward to, "I will be out there on such and such a date." Schedules were rearranged. We cherished every moment.

My husband belonged to a hunting club about an hour

north of us. Dad decided to come out this particular winter for a visit. We reserved the club and brought everything needed for a special time with my family and my sister's family. It involved much preparation: bed linens, food, games, literally everything. It just happened that there was a huge snowstorm. Dad kept looking out the window commenting that he did not see a plow and was getting concerned that we could not get out of there. We played it up to increase his concern knowing it was no problem. He had forgotten New York weather after living in California for so long. There was a giant fireplace. He loved putting on the logs and stoking the fire. Much fun and many unforgettable memories were made that weekend. The kids had fun with grandpa, and we totally enjoyed our dad. There was not a television and no distractions. God had done a thorough job and removed all of the past hurt from me regarding my dad.

During one of our visits to California, my sister and I were visiting with dad and his wife, Phyllis. Dad went to bed and Phyllis proceeded to tell us that when I was a baby, she and dad lived in Brooklyn. My mother came to their door and asked for money because I was sick. Phyllis then said, "You know, you were meant to be an abortion." Then she went to bed. Well, there we sat digesting that bomb! My sister finally said, "Well, God sure wanted you!" It was uncalled for and hurtful for Phyllis to tell me this. I did not really have a relationship with Phyllis though she had always been civil to me. A few times my dad had to shorten his visit out here when she called and said she did not feel well and wanted him to return to California. She knew he loved coming east to visit his first children, and I suspect she resented that.

I had been told by my mother's sister that I had a twin that died before birth. I assumed it was a miscarriage, therefore fraternal twins. So, now I know it was true. I had grown in my faith and in Jesus so I was not devastated. *But why would a mother try to kill her baby?* I wondered. How surprised she must have been to still give birth to me. My mother had five children very close in age. I'm sure it was overwhelming to anticipate another child with an absent father, no way of support and being mentally unstable.

In God's word, Psalm 139:13-16 says, "For You created my inmost being; You knit me together in my mother's womb. I praise You because I am fearfully and wonderfully made; Your works are wonderful, I know that full well. My frame was not hidden from you when I was made in a secret place, when I was woven together in the depths of the earth. Your eyes saw my unformed body; all the days that are ordained for me were written in your book before one of them came to be."

Psalm 22:10 says, "From birth I was cast on You; from my mother's womb You have been my God."

Because life is precious to Jesus, now I have a brother or sister in Heaven that I will meet someday. God's ways are not our ways, and I do not know why I was spared. But for His glory, I am telling my life story. For He has been in this at the very beginning bringing me to an understanding of Him. There is in Jesus, so much more than I can ever fathom. I never pursued this with my dad as I did not want to upset the relationship we had nurtured. In retrospect, I wish I had.

In God's mercy and during another visit to California, I was sitting alone again with Phyllis. I was led to share with her that Jesus loved her and died for her and if she asked Him to forgive her sins, He would come into her life and heart. She asked Him into her heart with tears rolling down her cheeks. That was a healing moment and one I shared with my eight brothers and sisters. God is love and loves everyone. He sees us just as we are and still loves us and forgives us. We just need to confess and ask. It has always been my desire that all fifteen of us children would one day be a family in Heaven.

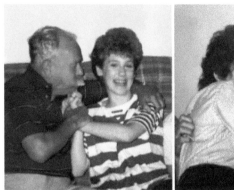
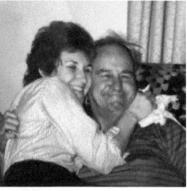

(Left) Never a dull moment! Dad pushing his false teeth out at Maureen (1987)
(Right) Snuggle time! Betty and Dad making up for lost years (1990)

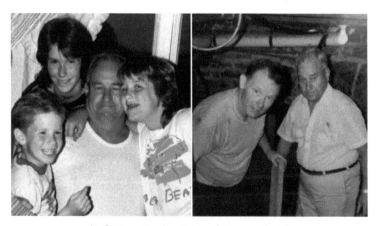

(Left) Dan, Carolyn, Dad and Maureen (1983)
(Right) Howard and dad working on an apartment house on Madison Street,
Glens Falls (1983)

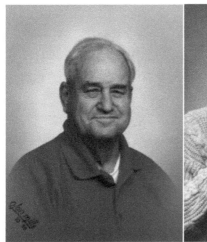
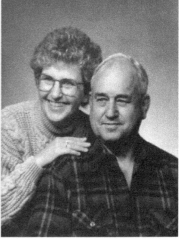

(Left) Dad (1991)
(Right) Betty and Dad (1991)

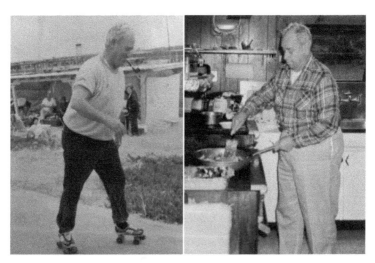

(Left) Dad roller skating in San Deigo, CA
(Right) "Chef" Dad cooking at the Niabi Hunting Club, North River, NY (1983)

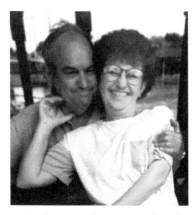

Dad and Betty Dad came to be there for
Carolyn's driver's education test. Glens
Falls, NY (1983)

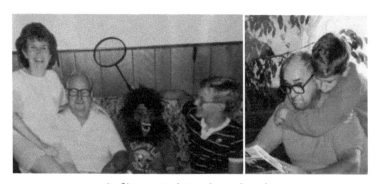

(Left) Betty, Dad, Brandon and Brodie
Brother Fred's house on Shoemaker Hill, Mohawk, NY (1984)
(Right) Dad and Dan (1985)

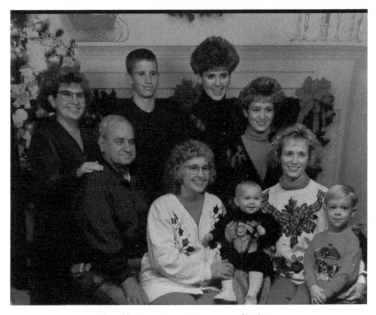

(Back) Betty, Dan, Maureen and Felicia
(Front) Dad, Madeline and Allison (Katie, Nathan children)
"Festival of Trees" at Queensbury Hotel (1993)

16

Scoliosis - A Mountain Too Big

Scoliosis : curvature of the spine

"He is my refuge and strength, a very present help in trouble"
(Psalm 46:1).

My middle daughter, Maureen, was now 13 years old. She was diagnosed with curvature of her spine, scoliosis. I faithfully took her for four years to my chiropractor who said she was getting better. That same year, she and a friend decided to diet and lose excess weight. As she lost weight, it was obvious to the naked eye that she had a serious curvature. My husband and I decided to take her to a scoliosis specialist in Albany, New York, an hour away. Finally, the day of the appointment arrived. We had no idea that our world would come crashing down. After his examination, in front of our daughter, he proceeded to say that Maureen had a 45-degree curvature. He said she needed surgery, rods, and should be wearing a Milwaukee brace *immediately*. In full detail he described the surgery, bringing our daughter to tears. "For God's sake, get help for your daughter," he said. *We were speechless!* His words were like a slap in our faces. We took very good care of our children and were certainly not negligent! He sent us to get her fitted for the brace; our precious daughter submitting with tears through the horrible ordeal. We were in shock; our healthy, happy girl now in an emergency situation. We sat at lunch, silent, perplexed, and overwhelmed, trying to grasp this fast diagnosis and its implications. There was no way we could go through any illness with this doctor. I prayed, not knowing where to turn. Her curve was way beyond the help of a brace, so my husband called the insurance company immediately and canceled it. My church family was praying for us and were a great support. There are areas in our lives that are more difficult to handle than others; mine was, "Don't touch my children." We had to give her to Jesus knowing He loved her more than us. Crying and in prayer, I gave my little girl to Him. I trusted Him with her, not knowing the outcome.

It was very stressful, a teaching of God's direction and faithfulness. I called one medical center and could not get an appointment for two months; that door closed. My husband talked to one of his teachers whose daughter was under treatment for a cancerous tumor on her leg at Boston Children's Hospital. He asked him to ask the doctor if he could recommend a doctor known for the treatment of scoliosis. To our amazement, relief, and God's plan, his daughter's doctor *was* the specialist.

Within two weeks, we had an appointment. I asked how many surgeries he had performed, not knowing that he was world renowned for his technique and taught in many countries. He humbly shared his information. God once again took care of His children with excellence. He directs our steps.

Surgery was scheduled in March 1984, three months from our first visit. We had much to do in six weeks. Maureen needed to donate six pints of her blood for surgery. In the 1980's, giving your own blood was not a common practice; it was called autonomous donation. The Lord had placed in my heart that Maureen was to have access to her own blood. To do this, I had to research to see how it could be done. It would not be done locally, but at the Red Cross in Albany, New York. From there they would ship it to the Boston Children's Hospital. She had to be able to give a pint a week to meet the deadline of surgery.

To submit your daughter who seems perfectly fine with no pain through this ordeal, was a difficult decision. The other option was to do nothing, but eventually she would suffer with heart and lung involvement. It had to be done. My faithful, Jesus, would bring us through this. I prayed.

Our first visit to the Red Cross was horrendous. Maureen had rolling veins and needed to be poked with a needle many times. Crying and shaking, she submitted to this knowing how important this was, even at 13 years of age. I was silently crying out to Jesus, *Why does it have to be like this? Why does she have to suffer? Where are you?* The first pint of blood was done. We also learned if she drank and ate before the blood draw, her veins would be filled and make the procedure easier. Because of that first visit, they made sure we always had the best nurse who found her vein easily. On her last visit, after five weeks, they tested her iron level. Unfortunately, it was low. She cried because she knew she needed one more pint. They retested and she was able to donate. She was so brave, so much for a young girl to grasp.

I realized why God had placed on my heart that she give her own blood for her surgery. In the news, it was announced that some donated blood was tainted with the AIDS virus. It was quite a stir in the medical community. I praised the Lord, for we would know she was safe with her own blood. This was just the beginning of this trial with Jesus. We did not want to go through this, but in our hearts we knew for her future, we had to walk this path with Him. My dad came for a visit just before surgery to be with Maureen. In his own way, he gave her a giant bear hug and said, "Kick 'em in the a--!" That was a way he could cover his emotions, too. He had a special place in his heart for "the Moose."

The day arrived; my stomach was full of butterflies. Courage is overcoming in the midst of fear. In our last meeting with the doctor, we had to sign papers acknowledging that we knew this surgery could cause paralysis or death. Maureen had to sign, too. It was a very sober time. *Oh, Jesus help! I know you are here!* I silently prayed.

We admitted Maureen, and she was placed in a ward with three other children, some with much more serious conditions than her. In those days they did not let you stay with your children. I woke up early, 3:00 a.m., to get ready and arrived at the hospital. They had given her Valium to quiet her nerves, but it had little effect. Maureen was quietly crying and quite anxious. I was trying to be brave for her. As she was being wheeled down the hall, we said our goodbyes. Howard ducked into a room and said, "Why are we doing this?" God gave me the strength and wisdom to know it had to be done. We would have loved to just bring her home, but in our hearts we knew better. We thought our goodbyes were done, but suddenly a nurse came back and said we could stay with Maureen until she went through those doors. Oh, it was so difficult and heart-wrenching. We had our trust in Jesus. *"Would we get her back? Would He take her home to be with Him?* Many concerning questions came to my mind. The long waiting began. In John 14:27, Jesus says, "Peace I leave with you, My peace I give you. I do not give it to you as the world gives. Do not let your hearts be troubled and do not be afraid." At this time I was anxious, but had an inner steadfastness that kept me from fear. I can face this in Jesus.

We were waiting in a special waiting room when the phone rang. A nurse said, "Mrs. Raymond, this is for you." My heart skipped a beat. The surgeon had called during the surgery to tell us they had just woken Maureen up enough to be sure she could move everything. Wow, imagine that! What a relief, but not a great vision of her on a table with her back open. *Thank you again, Lord*, I quietly said to Him. We had signed up for a trial of medications for pain control. Intensive Care was two days; someone was at her side full-time. She could only have ice chips, but pain control was great. Maureen was sent back to her room. It was then I really took notice of the other children. One had cancer, so much worse than scoliosis. The day arrived for her to stand. Wow, I was shocked! I was not prepared that she would be one and a half inches taller, for she was already tall! My husband had to return to work. I was alone in the big city of Boston.

Being left alone in a strange place was a big thing, especially with my history of panic attacks. But my Lord went before me. I had a room in a dormitory across the street from the hospital. It was private and one of a few with my own bath for $16 a night. I could easily make my way to Maureen's room through the Emergency Room entrance. I would cross stitch as she slept. I was there with her, where I wanted to be. She had been kept comfortable and progressed without a problem. We made it and thanked Jesus for every step, every advance, for everything: answered prayer, a $16 room with a bath, and for me, peace. It was all taken care of, directed by my Jesus: the hospital, doctors, the nurses, and insurance coverage. There was so much to be thankful for. This was a lesson in trust and resting in Him. *Teach Me, Lord*, I asked. I was able to focus totally on Maureen, free of anxiety, and full of joy.

Maureen was hospitalized for 10 days. I was able to be by her side the whole time. She was my miracle daughter, blessed by God. In the midst of this crisis, God gave us fond memories, special visits from loved ones, a different teddy bear every day, new friends, and experiences. We did good! *Let's go home*, I thought excitedly. We put an egg crate mattress in our minivan for the return trip. She slept and played music.

We were home at last with a body jacket and many directions. I looked, as she lay tucked in her own bed with our yellow lab, Suki, lying next to her. I gave her a good night kiss. Now to recover. *Thank you, Jesus*. I prayed with gratitude. I will continue to sleep in peace tonight knowing He is continuing to heal her back.

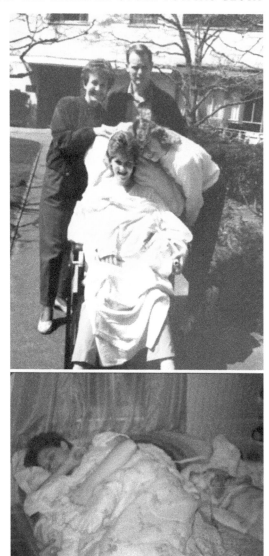

(Top) Betty, Howard, Maureen and Carolyn
Boston Children's Hospital (March 28, 1986)
(Bottom) Maureen and Suki dog back at home Vaughn
Road, Hudson Falls (April 1986)

17

Indecision: What About Mom?

Indecision: a wavering between two or more possible courses of action; wavering, vacillation

"Consider it all joy, my brothers, whenever you face trials of many kinds, because you know that the testing of your faith develops perseverance. Perseverance must finish its work so that you may be mature and complete, not lacking anything. If any of you lacks wisdom, he should ask God, who gives generously to all without finding fault, and it will be given to him" (James 1:2-5).

My mom was still in the nursing home in Sheepshead Bay, Brooklyn. My Aunt Grace, mom's sister, had just been diagnosed with advanced breast cancer. During my visit to her, I would visit mom in the nursing home. She seemed a little more alert and actually could carry on a short conversation. Aunt Grace was mom's main caregiver; she tended to all her needs, cigarettes, and all. I wondered who would be there for my mother if my Aunt Grace's breast cancer was fatal. Aunt Grace had received Jesus at a Billy Graham crusade and knew her eternal home was Heaven. The cancer progressed quickly and my sister and I found ourselves contemplating if we should bring mom to Glens Falls. *Where did that come from?* I questioned. I used to say my mother was dead. I was ashamed and humiliated by her illness, her nicotine stained hands, her appearance and her lack of communication. Do I want her in my town? How *selfish*! God had a lot of work to do. He had been working on my heart for me to even entertain the thought of bringing her here and including her in my life. I asked myself, *Do I dare try to get to know this woman with whom I had no real relationship? Do I take that wall down?* The Lord says in Proverbs 3:5-6, "Trust in the Lord with all your heart and lean not on your own understanding; in all your ways acknowledge Him and He will direct your path."

My sister and I took mom up to the sunny rooftop of the nursing home on one of our trips. We presented the gospel to her. We asked her, "Would you like to ask Jesus into your heart and ask forgiveness?" It was not a quick response. We waited, but then she decided. Yes! We quietly said the prayer, and she was now a born again child of God. Praise the Lord! After her decision and much paperwork, it was decided she would come to Glens Falls. *Did she want to?* I wondered. It was a big decision for her; leaving her routine, a life she was used to. She agreed, but it was a big decision for us and for her. Walking by faith is trusting in Jesus to lead you on His path for you. It truly was a time of desiring what He wanted. He knew what I needed more than I did myself.

We went to the Adirondack Manor, an adult home, in Glens Falls to ask if they would accept mom. There was no immediate decision. Medicaid had to be switched to a different county. Her mental issues weighed in their decision as well. We waited and waited. The Medicaid representative was making the transfer very difficult. Finally one day, the phone rang. "Mrs. Raymond, could you come to the Adirondack Manor?" A time was set. My sister and I listened to the director explain that she would not be an easy case, but they had decided to take her. Much to my amazement I burst out crying intensely, sobbing in emotional release. *Why was I crying? Did I need my mother?* I thought. It must be I wanted her here more than I imagined, or God wanted her here. Little did we know what the next two years would bring.

After much arranging, we picked mom up at Sheepshead Bay and drove the four hours home. How strange that must have been for her; how scary. She was also taking a big risk trusting us. Her room was ready at the Manor. We unpacked and settled her in the best we could. She had a roommate, but she kept to herself.

The first thing we did was organize a first-time get together with mom and her five children. My brother and sister came from California for this big, emotional first. All five of us had never been together, all at once with our mom - not that we could remember, anyway. We bought a beautiful dress for her, and we did her hair and nails. She was squeaky clean, like our mom should be. We had never celebrated birthdays, Thanksgiving or Christmas together. The excitement could be felt as we gathered together. But in the midst of it all, there was a sadness; a life which had missed it all, and all our lives too.

In one weekend, we had Christmas with a decorated tree, a big birthday cake for all of us, and a delicious Thanksgiving turkey dinner. Here we were all adults celebrating for the first time all these occasions that most take for granted. We had a professional photographer to immortalize this time together. The day was more for all of us, our need for a mother, the need to be loved, and the knowledge that we all had to accept our situation with the way life was with mom. How does that void get filled? Jesus. Papa God is love. He sees it all, and fills us with His love.

18

Life with Mom

Compassion: sympathetic consciousness of others' distress together with a desire to alleviate it

"My grace is sufficient for thee. For my power is made complete in weakness" (II Corinthians 12:9).

My sister Madeline and I had wonderful husbands and families which helped up us get through the difficulties of taking care of mom. It was a much more demanding commitment than any of us expected. Mentally, she needed to see my sister or me every day. There were activities posted, but she never would participate. We were the activity day in and day out. Mom had good days and bad days. She could smile and seemed content. All of a sudden, she'd get this "different look." She'd follow it by saying something like, "You will leave me flat," or something else strange.

The Manor had a great kitchen staff and would allow me to eat lunch or dinner with mom. We would play cards, look at pictures, and sometimes try to include my children for a visit. Those were long stretches of time and difficult to fill. It was easier to bring her home to enjoy a real home environment. I never wanted her to look like that unloved, homeless woman she was at the nursing home, so I did her hair and her nails. Her favorite color was blood red.

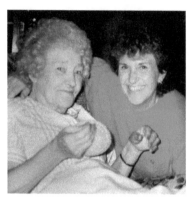

"Manicure by Betty" at Adirondack
Manor Bay Road, Queensbury, NY
(1989)

She was very medicated and had to take long naps. In nice weather, she would lay on my porch glider. I would tuck her in just like a child that needed the love and care. Mom related to my son, the youngest, and loved my big yellow Labrador Retriever. She especially loved to watch Dan from our enclosed porch as he kicked the ball or rode his bike. He was about nine years old, just the right age to enjoy this unusual Grandma, accepting easily this woman who smiled at him but said little. She always had a smile for Daniel and my dog. Life had been stolen from mom; five children and sixteen grandchildren. She was denied watching them grow up and being involved in their lives.

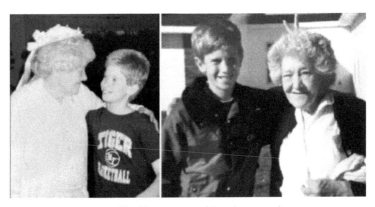

"Good buddies" Mom and Dan (1989-1990)

I tried to make it up to her. We canned tomatoes, cooked, listened to music, did various crafts, things that one would do in normal living. She did them, but not with enthusiasm. During the winter, she looked out at the snow covered trees and said, "God decorated those trees." This was so precious. She was a guest, a visitor in her life with us. It was actually a sacrifice for her to leave her routine and familiar surroundings of the nursing home. I had to realize that a real mother-daughter relationship was impossible. I was full of compassion and felt responsible for this lady called mom but knew we would not truly relate until we were in eternity. There was comfort in knowing that. My job was to be faithful and take care of Jesus' precious jewel, mom.

My sister and I each had three children, so we had to maintain their care, schedules, and keep life on an even keel.

It became very tiring even though we took turns. If it was a bad day for her, we shared the day.

Mom had a wonderful, caring, psychiatric nurse who recommended we send her to a place called Liberty House. This facility reached out to many with these variety of problems. Two or three days a week, a bus would pick her up and she could participate in various activities or just observe the hustle and bustle. We had to bring mom for an interview, and we were very thankful that they accepted her. We told her she was going to "school." Now on our day, we would go early before the bus pick-up and get mom very presentable and squeaky clean. At last we had free days to tend to our own homes and families. Now we only had to tuck her in at night. All this time was not without many issues, and the staff was gracious and worked through problems. Mom was a heavy smoker and required cartons of cigarettes; a carton a week, an expense we had to absorb.

One day the Manor called and said mom told her roommate, "I am going to murder you." The call arrived, "Mrs. Raymond, would she do this?" How did I know? She did take a knife to my step-grandfather when I was young. We picked her up and took her to the Mental Health Unit at Glens Falls Hospital, a place we said we would never go! Enter the inner sanctuary of mental illness and more medications. Back she went to the Manor. Her roommate was moved; praise God she could stay.

Yet another hurdle arrived. Shortly after, we were notified that mom was losing her Medicaid coverage. Well, I recognized this right away. I knew God would work it out. Our husbands could not afford this expense. Mom's psychiatric nurse went to bat for us at the hearing, where again, the story of our life had to be presented. Eventually, the coverage was reinstated. *Thank you, Lord, for your peace!* I cried out to Him.

One day, I had to run errands, but it was my day to have mom. I had her belted in the front seat of my van, and told her to stay in the car. "I'll be back in a few minutes," I said. Well, I returned to the car; No Mom!!! I was in a state of panic! I looked around, and then I saw her walking down the city street in front of our police station puffing on her cigarette in her nicotine-stained hands. Well, I burst out laughing. There she was, in the sight of everyone. This was my biggest fear ever; my mom walking on my streets. *Who cares? My mom was mom, and I was me. We were separate people*, I told myself. I did not have to be like my mom. I did not have to be ashamed of this woman. The lie my Uncle Frank often spoke over me during childhood, "You will be just like your mother," was exposed, and I was free. Freedom at last!!! God did a big work in my life and heart that day. Oh, how He worked things out just for me. Down came the walls of fear and shame. Freedom at last!!!

John 8:32 says, "And you will know the truth and the truth will make you free. Freedom comes by renewing your mind in God's word. His truth overcomes all the lies that have been a part of your mind." I had a sound mind!

1 Timothy 1:7 says, "God has not given me the spirit of fear but of love, power and a sound mind." I was settled in His love and word.

My brother's home was a two hour drive. We decided to take mom on a road trip with our six children to see them. This was a big step traveling with mom and visiting her oldest son and family. I thought I was doing this as something special for mom, but really it made me feel good. Mom had an institutionalized life. It was a life of routine, repetition, nothing unexpected, and simple demands. Off we went trying to pretend mom was enjoying herself. She started labored breathing at night and we had to travel 30 minutes to admit her to the hospital with congestive heart failure. Mom was not able, nor did she really want any adventures, just security and safety. We had a mom. But did we? I knew that God brought her to Glens Falls for me to deal with mental illness head on. It was not mom that I was afraid of, but mental illness: the destroyer of many lives and families. I wondered, *Could I love this woman that tried to abort me? Could I love with unreciprocated love?* Agape love, God's love, is free, not hinging on any return. God enabled me to forgive this lady. He helped me to love her to the best of my ability. I was able to love and accept her just as she was, despite not having many fond memories to draw upon. She was a mom of seven children who, because of mental illness, had a life which I had a hard time comprehending. I wanted to bless her, let her feel love and acceptance. God gave me and my sister the privilege of taking care of our mom.

My husband and I were planning a trip to Branson, Missouri for our 25th wedding anniversary. Mom was in the Adirondack Manor and my sister said she would fill in for me. I was scheduled for my regular mammogram and waited for the results. I received a phone call from the radiology department saying they wanted to retake the x-ray. Then, I received a call from my gynecologist suggesting I see a surgeon. Many times the doctors recommend that you wait six months for another x-ray. I am so thankful my doctor had God's wisdom.

I did not want my mother to know and kept her from the diagnosis and the treatment. For me I had been totally prepared by my caring and loving father, God. In the midst of mom, I was in my biggest miracle. I had been reading a book called, *In His Presence* by E. W. Kenyon, that I had bought at a garage sale years earlier. I just happened to start reading it (directed by Him). It was a faith builder with many scriptures. I had also attended a tent meeting when I only had the lump and asked for prayer for healing. The pastor prayed and said, "Through your illness, many will come to know the Lord." Well, I knew then that I had cancer, but I also knew that God was in it. The anniversary trip was canceled.

My husband and I were on a day trip and as I sat in the front seat of his truck, waves of fear started in my belly. I frantically thought, *How do I handle this? It was too big for me.* I started saying to myself, *"Greater is He that is in me than He that is of the world." 1 John 4: 4.* I did not know then that wave of fear was from our enemy, Satan. The word of God is powerful and Satan has to flee. After that episode, I was without fear, worry, and functioned every day without fearing the big "C." God allowed me to go through the whole process, but in it, the miracles abounded. During the biopsy I only wanted Novocain when they usually sedate you, and I also wanted to hear music. The next surgery was a lumpectomy. I was joking with the doctor as I had no pain from surgery, even after all my lymph nodes were removed. A liver CAT scan was part of my staging. It was a Friday, and the results showed a spot on my liver. I remember walking to the car, not at all upset, but thinking, *Well, I didn't think I was going to be Stage IV.*" I just had total faith and trust my Lord gave me. My husband and dad, who was visiting from California, were very upset. My husband called the doctor immediately so we did not have to wait the weekend for the results. The spot was a hemangioma, no problem. I just kept cooking dinner as my husband and family breathed a sigh of relief. God had given me the gift of faith. I could just put it all into His perfect hands; I could live or die, it was up to Him. I had to go through 40 radiation treatments, every day except weekends. The day after my last treatment, I flew to California. The doctor said I would be very itchy and have a reaction to radiation for I have a fair complexion. That never happened!!! I look back and wonder why this all happened. I flew through it all with no fear or stress. It was to show me God's love and strength, and that I am "the apple of his eye" just like He says in His word.

During this time, God gave me this scripture as a formula to get through all the trials of life:

> *Humble yourselves, therefore, under God's Mighty hand, that He may lift you up in due time. Cast all your anxiety on Him because He cares for you. Be self-controlled and alert, your enemy the devil prowls around like a roaring lion looking for someone to devour. Resist him, standing firm in the faith, because you know that your brothers throughout the world are undergoing the same kind of sufferings, and the God of all Grace, who called you into his eternal glory in Christ, after you have suffered a little while, will Himself restore you and make you strong, firm*

and steadfast. To Him be the power forever and ever. Amen. (1 Peter 5:6-11).

I was healed; that was 29 years ago. God can use doctors, medicine, or just outright healing from His hand. It is His choice, but we can be sure it is for our good. His promises are true, never wavering, and always "yes and Amen."

Then, the unexpected happened. The Adirondack Manor did not want mom any longer. Area nursing homes did not have any openings. She was placed on the third floor of the Glens Falls Hospital for one full year. This was a very trying, demanding time. Mom spent her days walking that one hall. It was so boring, day after day. This was a holding floor until placement; no activities, just bed, meals and medications. That was all. It was up to us to bring some joy and interest in her life. Thank God He had given me the ability to do crafts. I remember making wallpaper fans and decorating them, including other patients, as well. Taking care of the home front, children, their activities, and also meeting mom's needs became exhausting for me. Prayers were answered at last when mom was placed in a nursing home 20 miles away. It was an older facility, but finally mom had a bedroom with a real iron bed, scenery, and (almost) home cooking. My sister and I, once again, alternated days and usually would stop and pick up a treat like a sundae or a muffin.

Mom developed severe pain in her abdomen and was brought to the hospital Emergency Room. We insisted on an X-ray, and the doctor hesitantly ordered it. The X-ray showed she had a cracked pelvis; the pain was real. The pain took a back seat to her serious Chronic Obstructive Pulmonary Disease. Mom required much attention and care, and we stayed with her because she could not call for help for the necessary suctioning. It was evident that her days were limited on Earth. We tried to get help to keep her comfortable, but they would not increase her morphine. Mom died about a week later with a paid sitter, a friend, at her side. We know the death of His saints are precious in His sight, and an angel accompanied her home.

Mom's funeral was a celebration of her life. How can you celebrate this life of sorrow, pain, and what appeared as meaningless to others? She helped in the nursing home, and she pushed people around in wheelchairs. As for me, my mother developed my compassion, long-suffering and hope. She said she used to walk the hall praying for us. Did we really know the quality of her life? Any life is precious in God's sight and each life has a plan. Trust was an issue here. I thought, *Was I to dwell on how her life was or thank Him for the few years He gave her to me?* I chose to be thankful. When mom was laid to rest, Jesus had resolved many of my issues: fears, shame and rejection. Her friends from "school" came and many of my friends and family as well. Many testified how her life had touched them. On display were her many pictures with family and crafts. A friend played beautiful violin music, and my pastor delivered a great message.

1 Corinthians 12:18-27 states, "But in fact God has arranged the parts in the body, every one of them, just as He wanted them to be. If they were all one part, where would the body be? As it is, there are many parts, but one body. The eye cannot say to the hand, "I don't need you," and the head cannot say to the feet, "I don't need you!" On the contrary, those parts

of the body that seem to be weaker are indispensable, and the parts that we think are less honorable we treat with a special honor. And the parts that are unpresentable are treated with special modesty, while our presentable parts need no special treatment. But God has combined the members of the body and has given greater honor to the parts that lacked so that its parts should have equal concern for each other. If one part suffers, every part suffers with it; if one part is honored, every part rejoices with it."

In Ephesians 6: 2-3 it says, "Honor your father and mother which is the first commandment with a promise so that it may go well with you and that you may enjoy a long life on the Earth."

I honored my mom. She gave me life. Her life took a turn in a path she had never intended. By trusting Jesus and asking forgiveness for her sins, she is now in Heaven; whole, complete and at peace. After the funeral, the hospital chaplain came to us and suggested we come and talk to him. I am sure he felt we were not grieving as he thought we should. We were celebrating my mom's life and her homecoming to Jesus, not grieving for the life left behind. We had a good laugh! I thought, *How could you ever want mom back in her tormented state when we knew she was walking with Jesus?* He had no understanding there. I will see her again, totally normal and happy. Praise the Lord!

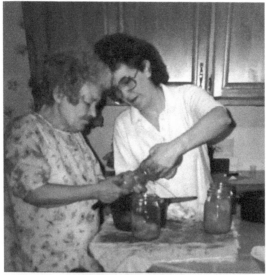

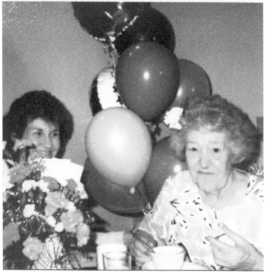

(Top) Mom and Betty canning tomatoes at Betty's home on
Vaughn Rd. (Bottom) Celebrating mom's 71st birthday at
The Adirondack Manor (1990)

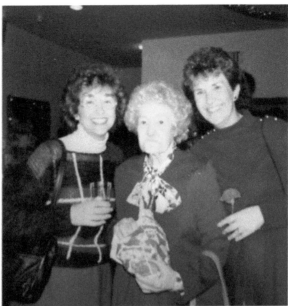

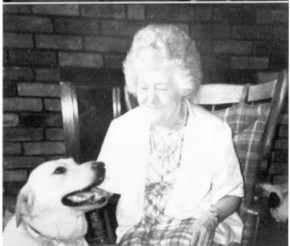

(Top) Madeline, Mom and Betty attending an activity at
The Adirondack Manor
(Bottom) Mom enjoying Soey the dog (1990)

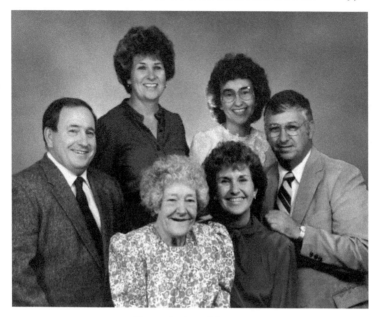

First gathering with mom
(Back row) Fred, Barb, Madeline and Ron
(Front row) Mom and Betty
Upper Bay Road, Lake George, NY (1989)

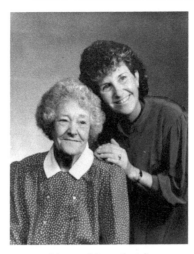

Mom and Betty (1989)

19

Dad's Last Visit

Restoration: re-establishment, the state or fact of being restored, a return to a former, normal condition, restitution of something taken away or lost

"And after you have suffered a little while, the God of all grace, who has called you to His eternal glory in Christ, will himself restore, confirm, strengthen and establish you" (1 Peter 5:10).

With anticipation, I looked forward to my dad's next trip. It was evident when he arrived that he was struggling to breathe. He had been diagnosed with asbestosis, a result of painting elevator shafts when he was younger. Even with this serious condition, he exuded joy, never heaviness. My son-in-law was a pastor at a small community church about forty miles away in Hague, New York. As Sunday approached, my dad said to him, "Preach me a good one, Mike." Mike had already prepared his sermon but felt led to give the salvation message. God sent His son for us because He loves us, and Jesus shed His blood on the cross to take away our sin. If we believed He was God's Son, confessed our sin, and invited Him into our heart and life, we would have eternal life. John 3:16 says, "For God so loved the world that He gave His one and only Son, that whosoever believes on Him should not perish but have eternal life."

My sister and I had presented the gospel to dad shortly after his first visit, and he said the prayer acknowledging his need for a Savior. After this message, he was assured of his salvation. He was safe in Jesus.

During this visit, he was able to attend my son's football game. This was a very important game and a very special time for both. It was a great visit, but his declining health was obvious.

Dad didn't like goodbyes. He would say goodbye the night before and quietly slip out the next morning with my husband on the way to the airport. This one morning I heard him, but respected his wishes and stayed in bed, pretending I was sleeping. He quietly came into my room and gently kissed my cheek and said, "Good-bye, baby girl." He left. Tears streamed down my cheeks. I needed the love of my earthly daddy. God is so good. He knows our needs and knows the gaps that need to be filled.

My God is a God of restoration. Yes, I had a part, as I submitted to His leading and faced the issues (the walls) that trapped me. He led me to restoration with my mom and dad. So many emotional issues, like a ball of yarn, to untangle: rejection, fear, depression, shame, inferiority, abandonment and insecurity.

That visit was in the fall. On Christmas Eve, I received a

phone call that my dad was in intensive care. I thought, *Should my sister and I fly to California while he was in the hospital or go to his funeral?* We prayed and both felt we should wait. We then heard that the airport would have been closed due to an ice storm. That decision was confirmed.

I called dad in intensive care to tell him how much I loved him. Oh, how I would miss these phone calls. When my sister called, he confirmed that "He did it," meaning he accepted Jesus as his Lord and Savior. He went to his eternal home shortly after. We flew to California for the funeral. Even my oldest brother flew out. My dad had 13 children. We had never been all together at the same time. At last we were able to be at this "Gentle Giant's" funeral to share the loving memories of his life. The service was conducted by a born-again Jewish pastor. Many of his children contributed during his service. The Lord had orchestrated the whole service. I had not had time to prepare anything to present about my dad, but had brought a devotional with me on the airplane. Within the many separate days, I found one devotion that was perfect for this time. It actually was the same one two of my siblings had shared with their families. My sister wrote a poem about dad and his children. The pastor led an altar call and some loved ones responded. It was a blessed time. As I gazed at my dad in the casket, this man I had learned to love, I thought that our God is so merciful. He had enabled me to forgive him and more importantly, he was totally forgiven by God because of Jesus' sacrifice. What an awesome God! My dad was now with Jesus celebrating his eternal home with many others. I can only imagine!

I still miss him and his ways, but mostly his love. He is

now in Heaven with mom, his second wife, Phyllis, and three of his children that have also since gone to Heaven. It's a different grief, sad, but not without hope. I will see him again. Praise the Lord!

Mom had said she walked the halls praying for her kids. She had missed out on so much. There was no replacing that on Earth. Her prayers were answered as all five of us know Jesus and have wonderful families. Each had to deal with the missing pieces in our lives.

We also wondered about our half-brothers, Jimmy and Paul. Long after mom went home to Jesus, we started searching for them. We were able to reach their father. Paul had committed suicide in Albany, and Jim lived in the state of Washington with his wife and four children. After a while, he flew out to meet us. He also knew Jesus; we rejoiced! He had mom's eyes. It was a friendly visit, and we occasionally stay in touch. God always knows in His love what is best for us.

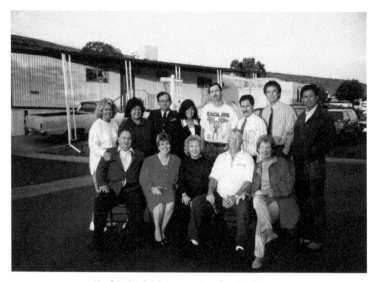

All of dad's children together for the first time
(Back) Phyllis Ann, Frances, Donald, Pat, Michael, Mark,
Steven and Phillip
(Front) Fred, Barb, Madeline, Ron and Betty
San Diego, CA (1996)

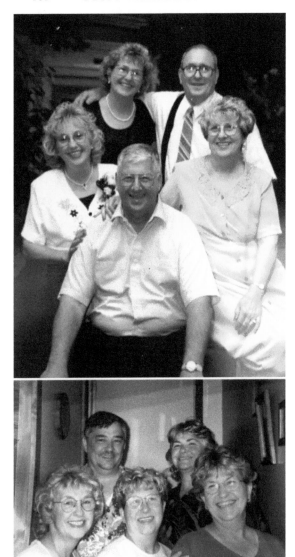

(Top) Betty, Fred, Madeline, Ron and Barb (1999) (Bottom)
Jim and his wife, Barb, Madeline, Barb and Betty. (1999)

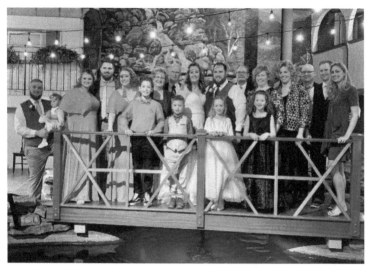

It's a wonderful life!! Our Granddaughter Sarah's Wedding
Betty and Howard with a growing family
(Feb. 22, 2020)

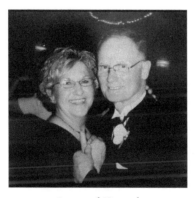

Betty and Howard
Maureen's wedding
Hiland Park Country Club,
Queensbury, NY (April 2007)

In Jeremiah 29:11-14 it says, "For I know the plans I have for you, declares the Lord, plans to prosper you and not harm you, plans to give you hope and a future. Then you will call upon me and come and pray to me and I will listen to you. You will seek me and find me when you seek me with all of your heart. I will be found by you and I will bring you back from captivity."

I was captive to fear, shame, inferiority, rejection, helplessness, hopelessness, insecurity, confusion and depression. I was a twisted mess, not knowing what to do. BUT, GOD DID!!!!!!!

At 27 years old, Jesus knocked on my heart and stepped into my life at the Billy Graham movie. I made my decision to accept and follow Him. He would do it, and I would follow. God's hand has been on me from the beginning, from my mother's womb; leading me, comforting me, changing me, healing me, and filling me with peace and joy. I have an abundant life and am blessed with a beautiful family.

Psalm 40: 2-3 says, "He lifted me out of the slimy pit, out of the muck and mire, he set my feet on a rock and gave me a firm place to stand. He put a new song in my mouth, a hymn of praise to our God." The enemy uses fear to steal our hope and limit our success. He uses fear as a weapon to stop us from reaching victory.

2 Peter 2:19 A says, "... for as a man is a slave to whatever has mastered him."

Jesus untangled my emotions, exposed the truth, and led me on the path to be healed. I had to deal with issues head on and let Him start the untwisting to make me whole. Yes, when I opened my heart and asked Him, I was promised eternal life. That promise started immediately and still encompasses everything.

John 10:10B says, "I have come that they may have life, and they would have abundance."

John 11:25-26 says, Jesus said to her, "I am the resurrection and the life. Whoever believes in me, though he die, yet shall he live, and everyone who lives and believes in me shall never die."

Today, is He knocking on your heart? Say, yes! It is the best decision you will ever make. He will take you out of that miry pit and set your feet upon a rock. Thank you, Jesus. John 3:16 says, "For God so loved the world that He gave His one and only son, that WHOEVER believes in Him shall not perish but have eternal life." *That "whoever" is you!*

Prayer of Salvation

Dear Jesus,

I confess that I need you. I ask you to forgive my sins. I believe you died for my sins and rose from the dead. I turn from my sins and invite you to come into my heart and life. Unravel the wounds of my heart, and make your home in me. I want to trust and follow you as my Lord and Savior, Thank you, Jesus. Amen.

WELCOME TO THE FAMILY OF GOD!!!!

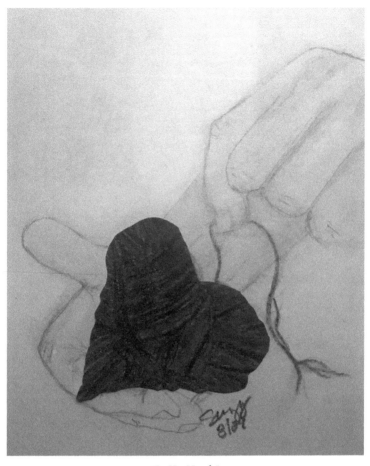

"In His Hands"
Drawing by Sue Colucci

The Dress

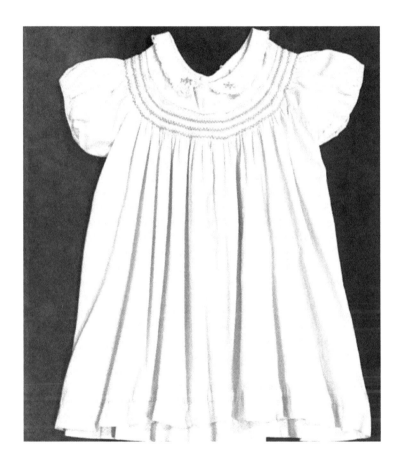

It's a miracle that with my tumultuous life, this dress is in my possession. This is the same dress you can find me wearing on page 4, in the photo of me and my siblings. I have this dress on display at my home. When I look at it, I am reminded of God's everlasting love and His hand of protection over me. This dress is more than likely a hand me down, which would make it over 77 years old. God is always in the details.

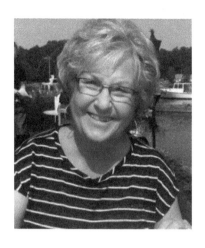

About Betty

Betty lives in the foothills of the Adirondack Mountains in Upstate New York with her husband of 56 years. She has three children, seven grandchildren, and three great-grand-children, which are all a joy! For 15 years, Betty led a support group for elderly women where she ministered to them through Bible study, homemade meals, crafts and adventures. She enjoys tole painting and participating in a yearly craft fair, *Christmas in the Country*. She is known for her cake decorating, cooking and making memories with her growing family. Her prayer is that many will find Christ after reading her story of His faithfulness and love. To contact Betty, please write to: behindthesmile777@gmail.com

CPSIA information can be obtained
at www.ICGtesting.com
Printed in the USA
LVHW070928310821
696554LV00014B/135